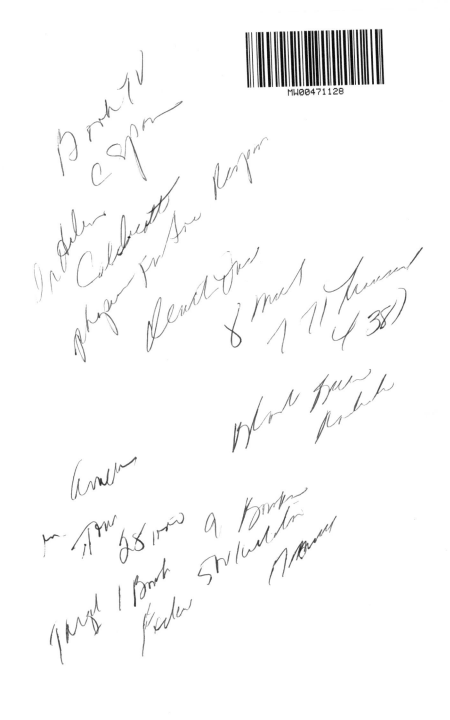

Lynda Madaras

TALKS TO TEENS ABOUT

AIDS

BOOKS BY LYNDA MADARAS

Lynda Madaras' Growing-Up Guide for Girls with
Area Madaras
The What's Happening to My Body? Book for Girls with
Area Madaras
The What's Happening to My Body? Book for Boys with
Dane Saavedra
The "What's Happening?" Workbook for Girls coauthored
by Area Madaras
Womancare: A Gynecological Guide to Your Body with
Jane Patterson, M.D.
Woman Doctor: The Education of Jane Patterson, M.D.
with Jane Patterson, M.D.
Great Expectations with Leigh Adams
The Alphabet Connection with Pam Palewicz-Rousseau
Child's Play

Lynda Madaras Talks to Teens About AIDS

AN ESSENTIAL GUIDE FOR PARENTS, TEACHERS, AND YOUNG PEOPLE

LYNDA MADARAS

Drawings by Jackie Aher

NEWMARKET PRESS 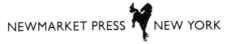 NEW YORK

This book is dedicated to the memory of Gregory Connell and to his mother, Mary Jane Edwards.

First Edition

92 93 94 FG 10 9 8 7 6 5 4 3   HC
92 93 94 FG 10 9 8 7 6 5 4 3 2 PB

Library of Congress Cataloging-in-Publication Data
Madaras, Lynda.
    Lynda Madaras talks to teens about AIDS.

Bibliography: p.
    Includes index.
    1. AIDS (Disease)—popular works.   I. Title.
RC607.A26M33 1988   616.9'792   87-31567
ISBN 1-55704-010-9 (hardcover)
ISBN 1-55704-009-5 (paperback)

Quantity Purchases

Companies, professional groups, clubs and other organizations may qualify for special terms when ordering quantities of this title. For information contact: Special Sales Dept., Newmarket Press, 18 East 48th Street, New York, New York 10017, (212) 832-3575.

Book design by Danzig/O'Bradovich

Drawings by Jackie Aher

Manufactured in the United States of America

CONTENTS

DIAGRAMS AND ILLUSTRATIONS

Until someone stands up and says this is a problem for the human race, that love and sex have been taken from our young, we're never going to win this battle.

Colleen Dewhurst
The New York Times
June 9, 1987

ACKNOWLEDGMENTS

Although there isn't space enough to list all of the individuals and organizations who assisted me in researching and writing this book, I would like to acknowledge the contributions of certain people and groups who were especially helpful.

Dr. Constance Wofsy, a leading AIDS researcher and a caring and compassionate clinician, was not only kind enough to write the preface and review this manuscript for medical accuracy, but also provided valuable non-medical insights. I am also greatly indebted to Dr. Donald Francis of the California Department of Health Services (DHS), who helped me understand the dynamics of this epidemic. Dr. Ken Kizer, Director of DHS, was likewise very generous in helping me find answers to my many questions about AIDS. Dr. Gerald Bernstein of the University of Southern Califoria (USC) was kind enough to share his expertise in the use of condoms and spermicidals in the prevention of AIDS. Dr. Everett Thiele devoted many long hours to helping me understand the statistical data and various math models developed to project the future spread of the epidemic. Barbara Lusey, an Outreach Worker with the Marion County Department of Health in Salem, Oregon, provided valuable information and insights about AIDS among IV drug users and addicted prostitutes. A number of other people and organizations assisted me in researching and preparing this manuscript, including Dr. Lawrence Mass, Paul Feldblum, Greg Daskalogrigorakis, Carol Vogel, Eva Lynd, Wallace Hamilton, Gillian Smith, and staff members at the Centers for Disease Control, the National Library of Medicine, the World Health Organization, and the USC Norris Medical Library.

My editor, Theresa Burns, made invaluable contributions to the overall organization of this book. And without the work of T. Carole Eden who helped with the research and also typed the bulk of the manuscript, this book quite literally would not have been written. I would like to thank Area Madaras, Evonne Pinto, Chandra Pinto, Jennifer Boggs, Janelle Mettler, the boys and girls in my sex education classes, and the numerous other teenagers who shared their concerns about AIDS and/or criticized parts of this manuscript for me.

Finally, let me note that their inclusion in these acknowledgments does not necessarily mean that these individuals agree with the opinions expressed in this book; and that I alone take responsibility for any possible errors.

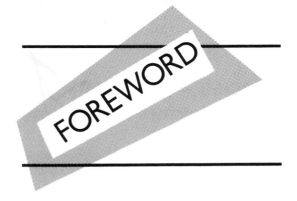

FOREWORD

As an infectious disease specialist on staff at San Francisco General Hospital, I began treating people with AIDS when the disease was first recognized back in 1981. Since that time, I have been actively involved in every aspect of the medical, social, and ethical policy issues surrounding the AIDS epidemic. I have cared for and counseled untold numbers of patients, given hundreds of talks, and worked with other researchers and policymakers at the city, state, and national levels. Both as a physician and as the mother of a ten-year-old daughter and a fourteen-year-old son, I have a special concern with educating young people about AIDS and its prevention.

Many parents have their own questions and fears about AIDS, which makes direct discussion of the topic with their kids difficult and embarrassing. And despite all the AIDS-related publications that have become available in the last few years, few have been targeted at teens. Thus, when I was asked to serve as a medical advisor for this book, I readily agreed. I'd received and was impressed by two other publications by Lynda Madaras, *The What's Happening to My Body? Book for Girls* and *The What's Happening to My Body? Book for Boys*. I was delighted at the prospect of a book about AIDS aimed at teens that used the same clear language and no-nonsense approach as these publications.

This book has met its goal. It is full of wise and practical advice, given in a way that teens can understand and use. Teenagers themselves share their personal experiences, some tragic, some funny, and all useful in getting important messages across. The medical information presented here is up-to-date and meticulously researched. The author has managed to take the wealth of information about this socially, medically, and ethically complicated disease and keep the tone simple, but accurate. It is the translation of complicated facts into everyday life and everyday language that makes this book so valuable. Kids can read it by themselves or with their parents. Parents would be well advised to read it themselves.

The style is matter-of-fact. There is no whining, no asking "Why did AIDS have to happen?" The author never points a finger, never lays blame. The message is "Okay, AIDS is here and we have to deal with it—here's how we can do it."

It is an important and much-needed message that Ms. Madaras puts forth in these pages. The teen years are years of experimentation—with approaches to sexuality, drugs, peers, ethics, and morals—as youngsters practice at being the adults they are going to become. Although the number of reported AIDS cases among teenagers is still quite low, teens are a potential next risk-group for AIDS. Yet, if they heed the practical wisdom in this book, and learn how to talk frankly to one another about this deadly disease, the current low teen-infection rate may well be maintained.

Today's teenagers are exposed to care-free sex on television at 8 PM, followed by an AIDS documentary at 9 PM, with a school report on AIDS due the next day. And the grown-ups who make the policies and decide what is "safe" didn't live through their own exhilarating, tortured, and self-conscious exploring teen years with the spectre of AIDS hanging over them. So, not surprisingly, many kids are tired of hearing about AIDS, or are distrustful of the information they get from grown-ups. But I believe that Ms. Madaras will win the trust and hold the attention of her audience, for she writes frankly and has a sense of what it means to come of age in the age of AIDS.

CONSTANCE WOFSY, M.D.
  Co-Director, AIDS Activities Division,
    and Assistant Chief, Infectious Diseases Division,
  San Francisco General Hospital

Talking to Teens
About AIDS:
a Preface for Parents, Teachers,
and Other Concerned Adults

Although the number of teen-agers with AIDS is miniscule compared with the 62,740 cases reported nationally, Margaret Oxtoby, medical epidemiologist for the CDC's AIDS Pediatric and Family Unit, said the number of teen-agers being diagnosed with AIDS each year is almost doubling and that the scale of the problem should not be underestimated.

Bob James
The Los Angeles Times
May 29, 1988

IN THE PAST, most teenagers who'd come down with AIDS were males, primarily hemophiliacs who'd gotten the disease from contaminated blood transfusions. Until recently, IV (intravenous) drug use was the major risk factor for teenage girls. But with the increase in the number of teen AIDS cases has come a change in the teen risk groups. Homosexual intercourse and IV drug use are now emerging as the major risk factors for adolescent boys. And the primary means of transmission among girls is heterosexual intercourse—in most cases, intercourse with a male IV drug user.

Although experts continue to debate whether the AIDS virus will ever become widespread among teens outside the risk groups, all agree that some such spread is inevitable. The fact that many teens belong to one of the high-risk groups and that there are 12 million sexually active teenagers in this country means *all* young men and women must be taught how to protect themselves against AIDS.

Imagine for just a moment that AIDS could spread by shaking hands. Parent and teachers would, of course, consider it their moral duty to educate teenagers about this deadly disease. Even if we thought it very unlikely that *our* sons, daughters, and students would get the disease, the fact that there was even a single teenage case anywhere in the country would be enough to convince us that our children needed to be taught about AIDS prevention. Indeed, parents and teachers would constantly be warning teenagers about the dangers of hand-shaking! If there were any reason to think that these warnings might be ignored, parents would tell their sons and daughters, "Look, I don't want you shaking hands, but if you're going to do it anyhow, I want you to wear gloves." And, in the AIDS prevention education courses that would be mandatory in all junior and senior high schools, teachers would not only provide instruction in the proper use of gloves, but would also distribute free pairs to all their students.

As you know, AIDS isn't spread through hand-shaking; it is primarily a sexually transmitted disease. But we mustn't let the fact that the disease is transmitted sexually keep us from teaching our youngsters how to protect themselves against this deadly disease. This book, which is aimed at the 14- to 19-year-old age group,will help you teach your youngsters the facts about AIDS and its prevention.

My Approach to Prevention Education

Since there has been considerable controversy over prevention education for teens, let me tell you a bit about my approach.

Abstinence

First, I explain that abstaining from sex until you're married or at least until you're older is an excellent way of reducing the AIDS risk. I also discuss other reasons for teenagers to abstain from sex and give advice that can help teens to stick to their decision to abstain. In addition, I explain that within the next couple of years we'll have the results of several important AIDS studies, which will give us a much clearer idea of just how widespread AIDS infection is and how much of a risk young people take by having sex. Thus, I tell teens that even if they wouldn't otherwise consider delaying sex, they should give serious consideration to the idea of abstaining from sex for at least the next year or so, until we know more about this disease.

Even if you didn't abstain from sex as a teenager or don't have moral objections of premarital sex, I hope you will reinforce the book's message that it's OK to say no to sex. All too often, the message our kids get from their peers and from the media is that there's something wrong with a teenager who isn't sexually active. So it's important for parents and teachers to let kids know that there is nothing wrong with choosing not to have sex.

Safe Sex Activities and Outercourse

Here I begin by telling teens not to make the mistake of thinking that sexual intercourse is the only way of being sexual. I then define safe sex activities—activities that don't involve the exchange of body fluids and, therefore, don't involve risk of AIDS transmission. And I explain that these activities are also ways of being physically close and intimate and of expressing love and affection. In addition, I present an alternative to intercourse known as outercourse. This involves sex activities such as mutual masturbation and is a way of having orgasm without any risk of AIDS (or pregnancy).

Given the fact that 12 million teens are sexually active and that we are faced with an epidemic of a fatal sexually transmitted disease, I think it's important for teens to know that outercourse is a safe alternative to intercourse. I hope parents and teachers will encourage sexually active young people to consider outercourse as an alternative to intercourse.

Practicing Safer Sex

For teens who are having sexual intercourse, this is a way to reduce the risk of AIDS by following three guidelines: 1) Limit the number of sex partners you have; 2) Choose your partners carefully; and 3) Use latex condoms when you have sex. I present this option to teens with lots of practical advice and all the nitty gritty details they'll need to know in order to follow these guidelines.

Here again, I hope you will reinforce the book's message that safer sex is only a meaningful method of risk reduction if *all three* guidelines are followed and that condoms alone do not provide enough protection. When condoms are used to prevent pregnancy, the failure rate is typically 12%, and it appears that the failure rate will be at least this high, if not higher, when they're used for the purpose of AIDS prevention. So make it clear that condoms alone are not enough and that teens must follow *all three* safer sex guidelines.

Please don't make the mistake of thinking that giving teenagers information about condoms will encourage them to go out and have sex. Many adults assume that if teenagers are given information about and access to birth control they will be more likely to have sex. But in the teenage mind, birth control and sex have only the most tenuous of connections. The average teen is sexually active for about a year before attempting to obtain a method of birth control. Even once they have a method, one-third use it only sporadically, and another third of sexually active teens never use contraception at all. Assuming that the availability of birth control causes sexual activity is putting the cart before the horse, at least by adolescent logic.

Moreover, if it were the availability of birth control that was causing teens to have sex, we wouldn't have over a million teen pregnancies each year. So don't let fear of encouraging sexual activity keep you from giving teenagers information about condoms.

I know there are some who feel that abstinence is the only morally acceptable means of AIDS prevention and that teenagers shouldn't be taught about safer sex. But this "abstinence only" approach ignores the fact that more than half of today's teenagers are sexually active and that fewer than 10% of couples are both virgins on their wedding night. As Elizabeth Whelan, a leading conservative, has said, "Our value system should not be so purist that it will condemn thousands of Americans to death." So, please don't jeopardize your teenagers' health by failing to give them complete information about all methods of AIDS risk reduction.

Better Red Than Dead—Some Tips on Talking to Teens About AIDS

Fewer than 15% of our nation's schools offer comprehensive sex education and, according to one recent survey, fewer than 10% of parents have ever had any really detailed, meaningful discussions about sexuality with their youngsters. But teaching teenagers about AIDS requires a very frank and explicit discussion of all modes of transmission, for as Surgeon General C. Everett Koop has so aptly put it, "You can't talk of the dangers of snake poisoning and not mention snakes." However, many of us can barely manage the birds and bees, let alone snakes! Please, remember, though, that nowhere is it written, "Thou shalt not be embarrassed." Fortunately, no one has ever actually died of embarrassment. Since the same cannot be said for AIDS, the bottom line here is that we have to forge ahead, despite our embarrassment. We really have no other choice. The following advice will help you talk to your teens about AIDS.

Don't try to pretend you're not embarrassed if, in fact, you are. Parents might say, "It's really hard for me to talk about this, but I don't want my embarrassment to keep us from discussing a subject as important as AIDS." Your child may adopt a maddeningly smug attitude about poor old, hung-up you. But grin and bear it—at least the two of you are talking about the subject.

Give kids "permission" to be less than totally all-knowing and cool. The unwritten rules that teenagers live by generally require maintaining an unwavering air of worldliness, especially in front of their peers. So, teachers in particular would do well to begin AIDS discussions by noting that the topic is an embarrassing one. (You might also add something like, "Maybe you've noticed that some people are so uncomfortable with this topic that, whenever it comes up, they immediately start cracking jokes or doing something to try and cover up their nervousness and embarrassment." This will effectively short-circuit the class clown who might otherwise have a field day here.)

First spend some time discussing sexuality, outside the context of disease. Please don't let the first words spoken about sex in your home or classroom be words about AIDS. "Sex is beautiful and wonderful, but it can kill you," is just not an appropriate way of introducing either of these topics. Once you've done that, you can then put your discussions about AIDS in the proper context by saying something like, "I want to talk to you about AIDS because I wouldn't want you to be harmed by something as wonderful as sex."

Appeal to your teenagers' sense of idealism and fair play. Explain that AIDS prevention is not just a matter of protecting yourself, but also of protecting others. You might say something along these lines: "I know you wouldn't want to do anything that was harmful to others. When you practice AIDS prevention, you are protecting others as well as yourself." Stress the fact that the decisions this generation of young people makes about sex and drugs may well determine the future course of this epidemic.

Explain your moral values, but don't moralize. You may or may not object to premarital sex. Your views on sexual morality may be based on religious beliefs, values such as respect for oneself and caring for others, or other personal convictions. Regardless of what your views are, it's important that you explain them to your children and discuss why you have these convictions. This is different from moralizing. One way to avoid moralizing is to use the pronoun *I* instead of *you* when talking to teenagers about moral values. For example, don't say, "You shouldn't do thus and such." Better to say, "I think that doing thus and such is a bad idea because . . ."

Tell them what love has to do with it. As one of my students once said, "Everybody talks about sex, but what about love? What's love got to do with it?" I use the poem printed below to start class discussions; you might want to read it to your teens.

What I Did Not Learn in Sex Class

in sex class
they taught us that
body temperature rises
during intercourse
they did not mention
the frozen isolation
afterwards
when love is not present

in sex class
they said touching is O.K.
you don't go to hell now
for sexual expression
it was not mentioned
that hell comes anyway
when minds and spirits
don't touch

we saw films
where they measured
responses
with wires and graphs
they did not teach
a way to measure
love
or the shock
of finding it was never there

Joy Sandulli Brown

CHAPTER ONE

AIDS: The Rumors and the Real Facts

THERE ARE A lot of rumors going around about AIDS these days. Some of the things people say are true, but some are only half true or even totally false.

RUMOR: *You can get AIDS from drinking out of the same glass or sharing food with an infected person.*

> FACT: This rumor is false. You can't get AIDS this way. Basically, people get AIDS by having sex with an infected person or by sharing needles used to inject illegal drugs.

RUMOR: *Teenagers don't need to worry about getting AIDS.*

> FACT: This rumor is only half true. Generally speaking, teens who don't use illegal drugs and who haven't started having sex don't need to worry about getting AIDS. But teens who are having sex or who do use these drugs *definitely* need to be concerned about AIDS.

RUMOR: *It's only when you have a certain kind of sex with certain kinds of people that you can get AIDS. As long as you don't have that kind of sex, you're safe.*

> FACT: This is false. The disease can attack anyone who is having any form of sexual intercourse or uses nee-

1

dles to take illegal drugs—regardless of where they live, what kind of lifestyle they lead, what race they belong to, or how old they are.

RUMOR: *AIDS is a killer. There's no cure and most people who come down with AIDS die within two years.*

FACT: This is true. Scientists have not been able to find a cure, and they aren't hopeful of finding one any time soon, if ever. Although it usually takes many years for people to develop any obvious symptoms, once they do develop a full-blown case of AIDS, most (75 percent) die within two years. No one has ever recovered from AIDS.

RUMOR: *If you know what to do, you can protect yourself against AIDS.*

FACT: This is true. AIDS can be prevented. People who learn the facts about AIDS prevention can help protect themselves against the disease.

With all the rumors that are going around, it's sometimes difficult to know just what to believe. That's where this book comes in. It will help you to learn the *real* facts about AIDS.

What Is AIDS?

AIDS is a very serious disease that affects the body's ability to defend itself against certain other diseases. The letters in the word AIDS stand for:

A—Acquired (something you get or develop)
I —Immune (the body's immune system)
D—Deficiency (a lack or a shortage of something)
S —Syndrome (a set of symptoms that can occur in people who have a particular disease)

Most scientists believe that AIDS is caused by a type of germ known as a virus. The virus has been given a number of different scientific names, including HTLV-III, LAV, ARV, and HIV.[1] Here in this book, though, we'll simply call it the AIDS virus.

The AIDS virus attacks and damages a part of the immune system, the body's built-in defense against disease. Because their immune systems are damaged, people with AIDS develop certain life-threatening illnesses that people with normal immune systems never get, or that they get and usually recover from quite easily. For example, people with AIDS may get:

Opportunistic Infections (OIs). These diseases can only strike because of the "opportunity" of the immune system that has been damaged. One of the most serious OIs is PCP (short for *pneumocystis carinii* pneumonia). This lung infection is caused by a germ that's all around us but that our immune systems easily keep in check. However, in people with AIDS, the germ multiplies rapidly, causing repeated bouts of PCP, which may eventually be fatal.

Rare Cancers. AIDS patients may develop rare forms of cancer, such as Kaposi's Sarcoma (KS), a cancer of the skin's blood vessels. Though rare and not fatal in other people, KS is common in AIDS patients and can cause death.

In addition to attacking the immune system, AIDS frequently infects brain cells, causing personality changes, inability to think clearly, and other serious mental abnormalities.

The Symptoms of AIDS

AIDS affects different people in different ways and may cause a wide variety of symptoms, depending on which diseases the person develops as the immune system breaks down. For example, if the person develops KS, there may be purple, blue, or pinkish spots on or under the skin.

For some people, the first symptoms resemble the flu or the common cold, except they tend to hang on longer and keep coming back. Some of the most common early symptoms are:

---

[1]HIV stands for *h*uman *i*mmunodeficiency *v*irus.

- swollen lymph glands in the neck, armpits, or elsewhere
- unexplained weight loss
- shortness of breath
- night sweats
- persistent, (long-lasting or recurring) fevers, headaches, cough, or diarrhea
- extreme tiredness
- unusual skin rashes
- white patches inside the mouth

Please remember that these symptoms may be caused by many other diseases. *Having one or more of these symptoms does not mean you have AIDS.*

Some people develop symptoms within a few weeks or months of being infected with the AIDS virus. But it typically takes five years or more for the symptoms to show up. Once people do develop symptoms, some become sick and stay sick until they die. But most people have periods of illness, then recovery, then illness, and so on until, finally, the immune system is so damaged that they can no longer recover.

AIDS patients may become very depressed and lose interest in life. In the last stages of the disease, some people seem to "waste away." There may be a loss of muscle control, inability to control urine or bowel movements, blindness, inability to speak or think normally, loss of memory, hallucinations, emotional outbursts, or other symptoms of mental illness. Some people lose their ability to walk or feed themselves. Some suffer great pain. AIDS can be a very horrible way to die.

AIDS vs. ARC

The letters ARC stand for *A*ids *R*elated *C*omplex. People with ARC are infected with the AIDS virus and have become ill or developed symptoms such as a swelling of the lymph nodes. But they don't have KS, PCP, or any of the other diseases you must have in order to be officially considered to have a full-blown, "classic" case of AIDS. People with ARC generally aren't as sick as people with AIDS; however, sometimes an ARC patient becomes seriously ill and even dies without ever having had a full-blown case of AIDS.

It is not known how many of the people who have ARC will actually go on to develop AIDS. Estimates are that about 20% will develop AIDS within 5 years; however, some experts believe that eventually, almost all ARC patients will develop AIDS. Like AIDS, ARC is incurable.

How People Get AIDS

The AIDS virus can live in a number of human body fluids, including blood, semen ("cum," the mixture of sperm and other fluids a male ejaculates during sex), and vaginal secretions (fluids made by glands inside the vagina). The AIDS virus can only be spread by direct blood-to-blood contact or close sexual contact with an infected person's body fluids.

The two most common ways of getting AIDS are by having sex with an infected person and by sharing IV (intravenous) needles used to take illegal drugs. Though it is much less common, AIDS can also be transmitted (passed from one person to the next) as a result of infected blood transfusions or infected women passing it on to their babies during pregnancy or childbirth.

Let's take a closer look at each of the methods of transmission.

Sexual intercourse. Most people who've come down with AIDS get the disease as a result of having sex with an infected person. You may have heard that only certain types of sexual intercourse can spread the disease, that a person has to have an open sore or irritation on the sex organs in order to get it, or that females can't pass it to males. These things are not true! *Any* type of sexual intercourse with an infected person may be capable of transmitting the disease, regardless of whether or not there's any sore or irritation. Moreover, females as well as males can pass the disease to their sex partners. (Chapter 2 will tell you more about sexual transmission.)

Sharing needles used to take illegal drugs. Sharing IV (intravenous) needles is the second most common way in which AIDS is transmitted in this country. When a person "shoots up" (injects illegal drugs), some of his or her blood remains in the needle and syringe. Thus, IV drug users who share needles or syringes that have been used by an infected person can get AIDS.

You can't, however, get AIDS from the needles used by nurses, doctors, dentists, or other healthcare workers because these people use disposable (throw-away) needles or ones that have been properly sterilized, i.e., heated or treated with chemicals to destroy any germs. (See Chapter 4 for more on needle transmission.)

Transfusions of blood or blood products. People have also gotten AIDS from having transfusions of blood or blood products (substances derived from blood). Such transfusions may be given before, during, or after an operation, if a person has lost too much blood. They are also used to treat certain diseases. For instance, transfusions of a blood product called "clotting factor concentrate" are used to treat *hemophilia*, a condition in which the blood does not clot properly and which can lead to uncontrollable internal (inside the body) bleeding.

If the blood or blood products used in a transfusion were donated by a person infected with AIDS, then the person receiving the transfusion may get AIDS. Because the blood product used to treat hemophilia is made from the blood of hundreds of different donors, many hemophiliacs have become infected with AIDS.

However, since 1985, all blood and blood products are carefully tested for AIDS before they are used in transfusions. So nowadays, there's very little chance of becoming infected with AIDS in this way. It's important to remember that *there's never been any danger of getting AIDS from donating, that is, from giving, blood.* The needles and equipment used to collect donated blood are disposable. They are only used once and then are thrown away, so there's no chance of becoming infected from donating blood. (See Chapter 4 for more on transmission through blood transfusion.)

Babies born to infected mothers. Infected pregnant women can pass AIDS to their babies before or during birth because the baby's and the mother's blood are in contact at these times. (See Chapter 4 for more on mother-to-infant transmission.)

You Don't Get AIDS From . . .

Unlike some viruses, the AIDS virus can't infect food or drinking water and isn't transmitted by insects or animals. Unlike the cold or flu virus, the AIDS virus doesn't live *in* the air or *on* the objects people touch. So, you don't get AIDS from what doctors call "casual contact."

YOU DON'T GET AIDS FROM:

- Cough or sneeze droplets in the air
- Holding hands, hugging, touching, being around someone with AIDS, or touching things an infected person has used
- Silverware, glasses, drinking fountains, towels, washcloths, doorknobs, or any of the other things people touch
- Swimming pools, hot tubs, showers, locker rooms, bathtubs, or toilet seats
- Normal, everyday activities like working in an office or attending school
- Eating in a restaurant, using a public bathroom, being in a crowd, or any other type of casual contact

The AIDS virus doesn't survive outside the human body fluids mentioned above. The virus doesn't enter the body through the lungs or digestive tract and it can't pass through unbroken outer skin. AIDS is a "blood-borne" disease. This means that the AIDS virus can only invade the human body by entering a person's bloodstream. In years of studying thousands of cases, no one has proven that even a single case of AIDS has been caused by casual contact.

How Can They Be So Sure AIDS Isn't Transmitted Casually?

Because it can take five to eight years or even longer for the symptoms to show up, people often wonder how scientists can be so sure that no one has gotten AIDS through casual contact. After all, isn't it possible that people really have become infected in this way, but no one's aware of this fact because there hasn't been enough time for these people to have developed symptoms yet? This is a good question, and one that bothers a lot of people. But there's a good answer.

Although it's true that it can take years for the symptoms to develop, there are certain tests (as we shall see later) that can tell us—usually within, at most, a few months—whether a person has been infected with the AIDS virus. Scientists have studied doctors, nurses, other healthcare workers, and family members of AIDS patients by means of these tests. Over a period of many months, or in some cases years, repeated tests have been given to people who'd never had sex with an infected person, used IV drugs, or had blood transfusions, but who had lived with or cared for AIDS patients. Many such people (thousands, in fact) have been tested for AIDS, and *none* have become infected through casual transmission.

There are a small number of healthcare workers who have become infected with the AIDS virus as a result of unusual accidents at work. In most cases, these were "needlestick" accidents, in which healthcare workers stuck themselves with needles that had been used to take blood from AIDS patients. We'll talk more about these healthcare workers in Chapter 4, but for now you should know that *none of these people became infected by casual transmission.* (P.S. If you still have unanswered questions about how AIDS is spread, don't worry—we'll get to them in Chapters 2 and 4.)

Exposure/Infection/Disease

You'll understand AIDS much better once you understand the difference between coming in contact with a virus, becoming infected with a virus, and actually developing a viral disease.

- *Exposure* means you've come into physical contact with the virus. Exposure may or may not lead to infection.

- *Infection* means the virus has moved inside the cells of your body. Once you're infected, you are usually capable of transmitting the virus to others. But being infected doesn't necessarily mean that you will develop symptoms and come down with the disease.
- *Disease* means you've actually developed symptoms. In other words, you "have" the disease; you've "come down with a case of" the disease.

Exposure to the AIDS virus. Not everyone who's exposed becomes infected. For example, many of the husbands, wives, and other long-term sex partners of people with AIDS have been exposed over and over again without becoming infected. Yet, there are also some people who have become infected after having sex with an infected person just once. Scientists don't know why some people exposed to the AIDS virus become infected and others don't.

Infection with the AIDS virus. If a person does become infected, he or she is capable of passing the virus on to others (e.g., through sex or sharing an IV needle). With most viral diseases, your immune system produces substances called antibodies that are designed to destroy that particular virus. Thus, your immune system eventually gains the upper hand and defeats the virus, so that you are no longer infected and can no longer infect others. But with the AIDS virus things do not proceed normally. The immune system can't defeat the AIDS virus (perhaps because the virus attacks the immune system itself). Antibodies are produced, but they aren't able to destroy the AIDS virus. Because there isn't a cure for AIDS and because the antibodies are ineffective there's no way to rid the body of the virus. So, it appears that people who become infected will stay infected for life. And we have to assume that they are also capable of infecting others for the rest of their lives. (In fact, there is some evidence to indicate that the longer people are infected, the *more* capable they are of infecting others.)

A person who's infected but doesn't yet have symptoms is called an *asymptomatic carrier* (*a* means "without"; *symptomatic* refers to symptoms). Such a person may or may not develop symptoms. (Remember, being infected with the

AIDS virus doesn't necessarily mean that a person will actually develop symptoms.)

Having the disease. Some of those who become infected do develop symptoms and actually come down with AIDS or ARC. Some people develop symptoms fairly quickly. But so far, the average time it takes to develop symptoms is eight years, and it may turn out that some people don't develop symptoms for 15 years or longer.

Experts have been estimating that at least 25% to 50% of those who become infected with the virus will develop AIDS within 5–10 years. Recent studies suggest that, as more time passes, this percentage may be much higher. Some experts now think 75% to 90% or more of those who become infected with the AIDS virus will eventually come down with the disease.

AIDS Antibody Tests

Scientists are trying to develop a reliable, inexpensive test that can tell if there are actually any AIDS *viruses* in a person's body. But currently the only test that can detect the virus itself is costly, complicated, takes a long time, and is only used for research purposes. However, we do have AIDS *antibody* tests.

Although AIDS antibody tests can't detect the virus itself, they can detect the antibodies that the immune system makes when a person becomes infected by the AIDS virus. If the test shows that the person has such antibodies, then the test is *positive*. A positive test means that, at some time in the past, the person became infected with the AIDS virus, and presumably still is. As I explained in the last section, with other infections the immune system eventually gains the upper hand; however, it doesn't seem to be able to defeat the AIDS virus. Since the AIDS antibodies made by the immune system can't destroy the virus, presumably the virus remains in the body. Therefore, a positive AIDS antibody test is considered a sign that the person is infected and is capable of passing the infection on to others. A positive test doesn't, however, mean that the person is actually going to come down with AIDS. (Remember, infection doesn't always lead to disease.)

If there aren't any AIDS antibodies in the person's blood, the test is *negative*. And as long as the person hasn't had any possible exposure to the AIDS virus in the previous six months (no IV drug use, no intercourse), then a negative test generally means the person isn't infected. However, if the person has done anything that could have exposed him or her to the virus in the six months before the test, it is possible that the negative result is a "false" negative. In other words, even though the test result was negative, the person really *is* infected. This can happen because it takes a while for the body to build up enough antibodies to show up on the test, usually about four to twelve weeks, but sometimes as long as six months.

A Cure, Treatment, or Vaccine

Scientists aren't hopeful of finding a cure for AIDS any time soon, if ever. For one thing, AIDS is caused by a virus, and medical science hasn't been able to find a cure for the common cold, herpes, polio, or any other viral diseases. Because of the way viruses reproduce (by taking over another cell's reproductive equipment) you can't kill a virus without killing the cell it has infected. The fact that the AIDS virus infects cells of the immune system and brain makes a cure unlikely, for killing these vital cells is simply out of the question.

Scientists are more hopeful of finding a drug treatment, one which can slow down the rate at which the virus reproduces. This could enable people to live longer, perhaps even to have normal lifespans. However, a major problem here is that in order to get to AIDS viruses that have infected brain cells, the drug must be able to cross the "blood-brain barrier" (a sort of filter that protects the brain from most germs). We don't have many drugs that can do that. Moreover, the drug would have to be powerful enough to slow down the AIDS virus, but mild enough so it doesn't harm the brain cells (a *very* tall order). Even if such a drug is found, there's still the problem of restoring the immune system. For these reasons, scientists don't expect to have an effective treatment any time soon.

Scientists are also working hard to develop a vaccine that could prevent people from becoming infected in the first place—the way the polio vaccine protects against polio. But experts say that it will be many years before an AIDS vaccine could possibly be ready. Even if scientists manage to speed up the normally long task of finding and testing a vaccine, it may turn out that it's simply not possible to develop an AIDS vaccine. For one thing, there are many different "strains" (variations) of the AIDS virus, and a vaccine that works against one strain of a virus often doesn't work against another. Also, vaccines work by stimulating the immune system to make antibodies against a particular germ. That way, if the germ ever enters the body again, the antibodies will be ready and waiting to destroy it. Unfortunately, the AIDS antibodies made by people's immune systems aren't able to kill the AIDS virus. Unless a vaccine can stimulate the immune system to make more effective antibodies, the AIDS vaccine simply will not work.

Because of the many problems involved in finding a cure, effective treatments, or a vaccine, preventing people from becoming infected in the first place appears to be our only way of stopping AIDS. In later chapters, we'll be talking more about prevention and what you can do to protect yourself against AIDS. But first you need to understand more about the spread of AIDS and who's most likely to get the disease.

The AIDS Epidemic: Origins and Worldwide Spread

Epidemic means "widespread" and the term definitely applies to AIDS. Cases of AIDS have been reported in over 100 countries and the World Health Organization (WHO) estimates that, worldwide, there are five to ten million people carrying the AIDS virus.

No one knows exactly where the AIDS virus came from, but many scientists think it originated in Africa. One theory is that the AIDS virus evolved from a similar, though harmless, virus found in the African green monkey. According to this theory, at some time in the past, one of the monkey viruses underwent a chance mutation[2] that enabled it to survive in the human body. This mutation was passed on to the virus's "offspring," and eventually some of these mutated viruses found their way into the human body, perhaps as a result of a person being bitten by or eating a monkey. (Monkey brains are a popular food in that part of the world.) Once inside the human body, the virus may have mutated further until it became the virus we know today as the AIDS virus. (Recent viruses that could be a sort of missing link between the monkey and AIDS viruses have been found in the blood of some Africans.)

Regardless of exactly where it started, AIDS is now a worldwide problem. It is most common in Central Africa and Haiti, but is also widespread in the U.S.

AIDS was first recognized here in this country. In the spring of 1981, the first five cases were reported to the U.S. Center for Disease Control (CDC).[3] The number of cases grew at an alarming rate from those first five cases in 1981, to nearly 50,000 cases by the end of 1987. And this figure only includes the people who've actually come down with a full-blown case of AIDS. An even larger number of Americans have ARC, or are infected but don't yet have symptoms. The CDC estimates that, as of the end of 1987, there were about one-and-a-half million asymptomatic carriers in the United States. Many experts feel that the CDC figures are too low and that as many as three million Americans may already be infected (see Illustration 1).

Because most of the people who are currently infected

---

[2]Although no one knows why it happens, we do know that, from time to time, all living things undergo chance mutations that make them slightly different from the others of their kind. Just as human beings evolved from apes, so all life forms on this planet evolved from some earlier form through this process of mutation. While mutations are fairly common, the particular type of mutation that could have resulted in the monkey virus evolving into the AIDS virus is very unusual.

[3]The CDC is a branch of the U.S. Public Health Service and is in charge of keeping track of diseases and any new epidemics in this country.

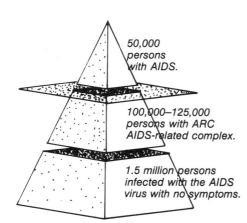

50,000 persons with AIDS.

100,000–125,000 persons with ARC AIDS-related complex.

1.5 million persons infected with the AIDS virus with no symptoms.

By the end of 1987, the CDC reported that nearly 50,000 Americans had AIDS, but this figure only included those who had full-blown cases of AIDS.

Experts estimate that at least 50% of the people with ARC will go on to develop AIDS within 10 years.

Many experts believe that eventually 90% or more of those infected with the virus will develop AIDS. Unless a cure is found, most or all of those who do will die.

Illustration 1. AIDS: The Hidden Epidemic The reported cases are only the "tip of the iceberg." The CDC estimates that for each reported case there are an additional 30 Americans who have ARC or who are infected with the AIDS virus but don't yet have symptoms. And some experts say the ratio is much higher than 30 to 1, perhaps 50 or even 100 to 1.

with the AIDS virus don't yet have symptoms, they may not even be aware of the fact that they are infected. But they are still capable of passing the disease on to others. So, every day more and more people are becoming infected. The CDC predicts that by 1991 the total number of cases in the United States will have reached at least 270,000. The World Health Organization (WHO) estimates that by 1991 the total number of actual AIDS cases *worldwide* may top three million, and that as many as *100 million people could be infected with the virus by 1991.*

AIDS Is Not a "Gay" Disease

Gay is a slang term for homosexuals. Despite what some people think, AIDS is not just a disease of homosexual or bisexual men; heterosexuals also get AIDS.

Since we'll be talking about these different types of sexuality throughout this book, let me say a few words about the meaning of these terms. *Homo* means "same" or "alike" and *hetero* means "opposite" or "different." The term *homosexuality* is used to describe romantic or sexual feelings, fantasies, crushes, or actual sexual experiences that include someone *of the same sex* as you are. When it's someone *of the opposite sex*, the term is *heterosexuality*.

Few of us are strictly homosexual or heterosexual in the sense that most people (about 90% of us) have a mixture of a hetero- and homosexual feelings. Having a few homosexual experiences *does not* mean that you're a homosexual. This is most common during the teen and pre-teen years and has nothing to do with whether you'll be a homosexual when you are grown up. Generally speaking, we consider a person to be a *homosexual* only if, as an adult, that person's strongest sexual attractions and most of his or her sexual activities involve someone of the same sex. (*Lesbian* is another term for a female homosexual.)

If an adult is most strongly attracted to the opposite sex, then he or she is considered a *heterosexual*. Men and women who are strongly attracted to both sexes and whose sexual experiences are about equally divided between partners of each sex are considered *bisexuals*.

The first cases of AIDS reported in the U.S. occurred in gay men, and the majority of Americans who've come down with the disease since then have also been male homosexuals or bisexuals. But it's a mistake to think of AIDS as a "gay disease." For one thing, American heterosexuals can and do get AIDS, both in sexual and nonsexual ways. Moreover, in Central Africa, where the disease is most widespread, virtually all the sexual transmission is between heterosexuals, either from male to female or vice versa. Although AIDS is most common among homosexuals in America, *on a worldwide scale AIDS is primarily a disease of heterosexuals.*

AIDS Risk Groups in the U.S.

When a disease is more common among certain groups of people, those groups are called risk, or high-risk, groups for that disease. The pie chart in Illustration 2 gives a breakdown of the adult and teen AIDS cases reported to the CDC as of May 2, 1988. (Children under 13 account for only about 1% of U.S. AIDS cases and are not included in Illustration 2.) It's important to remember that this chart includes only full-blown cases of AIDS and does not include people who have ARC or who are infected with the AIDS virus but have yet to develop any symptoms. It usually takes five to eight years or more for an infected person to develop a full-blown case of AIDS, which means that looking at today's cases can give us an idea of who was spreading the virus several years ago. But it doesn't tell us how widely the virus has spread since then, who's being infected today, or who will become infected in the future.

Doctors are required by law to report all patients with full-blown cases of AIDS to the CDC. Based on information provided by the doctor and/or the patient, the CDC assigns

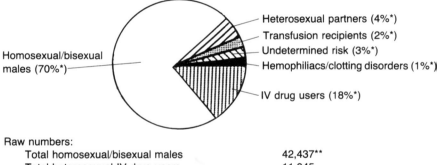

Heterosexual partners (4%*)
Transfusion recipients (2%*)
Undetermined risk (3%*)
Hemophiliacs/clotting disorders (1%*)
IV drug users (18%*)

Homosexual/bisexual males (70%*)

Raw numbers:

Total homosexual/bisexual males	42,437**
Total heterosexual IV drug users	11,045
Total hemophiliac/clotting disorders	591
Total heterosexual partners	2,463
Total transfusion recipients	1,467
Total undetermined risk	1,894
Total adult and teen cases	59,897

*These percentages have been rounded off, and therefore will not total exactly 100%.
**This includes 4,438 homosexual IV drug users.

Illustration 2. A Breakdown of U.S. AIDS Cases As of May 2, 1988, 59,897 adult or teen cases of AIDS had been reported to the CDC. This diagram shows the portion of cases attributed to each risk group.

the case to one of the risk groups. If the case doesn't fit into one of the risk groups, it's listed as "undetermined risk." If a case fits more than one group, the case is assigned to the group that comes first on the list. For example, a male homosexual who used IV drugs would be listed in the "homosexual/ bisexual male" group, not the "IV drug risk" group. The various groups on the list are described below.

Homosexual/bisexual males. As you can see, this is by far the largest of the U.S. AIDS risk groups. The majority of the men in this group are white, middle-class males who live on the east or west coast. However, there are men from all races, all economic levels, and all parts of the country in this group. About 7% of the men in this group are also IV drug users. One thing you should keep in mind is that the CDC lists any male with AIDS who's had sex with another male *even once since 1977* (believed to be the first year the virus began to spread in the U.S.) in this risk group.

IV drug users. This is the second largest U.S. risk group for AIDS, and includes male and female heterosexuals who've used IV drugs even once since 1977. (Homo- or bisexual males who use IV drugs are listed in the above group.) Many of the women in this risk group are also prostitutes (people who have sex for money). IV drug use is more common among men than women and is most common among males living in inner-city, poverty-stricken neighborhoods, which in the U.S. tend to be black or Hispanic communities. So, not surprisingly, the majority of people in this risk group are poor, urban, minority males. But here again, there are people from all races, all economic levels, and all parts of the country in this group.

Hemophiliac/clotting disorders. The people in this group have hemophilia or another of the similar, but even rarer, clotting disorders. Since most of the people in this group are hemophiliacs and since most people who suffer from hemophilia are males, most of the people in this group are males.

Heterosexual partners. The majority of people in this group are heterosexuals who do not fit into one of the above groups, but who have had sex with someone known to have AIDS or someone in one of the other risk groups. Since most of the people who now have AIDS are males, most of the heterosexual partners in this group are, of course, females. Although some of the females in this group got AIDS from a male bisexual or transfusion recipient, the majority got it from a male IV drug user. This group also includes heterosexuals who've come from Haiti, Central Africa, or any other place where AIDS is widespread among heterosexuals and who've entered the U.S. since 1977.

Transfusion recipients. This group includes people with AIDS who have received transfusions of blood or blood products, but who do not have hemophilia or any of the other clotting diseases. For some unknown reason, the majority of people in this group are also males.

Undetermined Risk. This includes a) male and female heterosexuals who don't fit into any of the other groups; b) people who had died before they could be questioned or were otherwise unable or unwilling to give information; c) people whose cases the CDC is still in the process of investigating; and d) one healthcare worker who developed AIDS after a needlestick accident (see pages 85–86).

Heterosexuals Outside the Risk Groups Are Not "Safe" From AIDS

"I'm not thin," says Marie, a 34-year-old office worker. "I'm not pale. I'm middle class. I'm heterosexual. I live in Kansas City. And I have AIDS."

She is sitting in the living room of her comfortable suburban housing complex with another woman, an AIDS counselor. "You're not supposed to have AIDS in Kansas City," agrees the other woman.

Marie's got two teenage kids, and she's been divorced for 15 years. During that time she's had just four sexual encounters. "I have not been a loose woman," Marie says, blushing. "I'm not a bar person and I haven't done drugs. I'm somebody's mother. Somebody's sister. Somebody's daughter. They say I'm in a low-risk group, so if I can get AIDS, anyone can."

People magazine, August 3, 1987

Cases like Marie's are very unusual. But Marie's story does show that heterosexuals who don't belong to an AIDS risk group can and do get AIDS. Will there be a lot more cases like Marie's in the future? Or will cases like Marie's only account for a small portion of the AIDS cases in the United States?

No one knows the complete answers to these questions. But the next chapter, which explains more about the sexual transmission and spread of AIDS, will help you to understand what is known about it. And as you'll learn in that chapter, everyone who is having sex or who plans to someday needs to know the facts about AIDS prevention—regardless of whether they belong to an AIDS risk group.

CHAPTER TWO
The Sexual Transmission and Spread of AIDS

SEXUAL TRANSMISSION IS the main means of spreading the AIDS virus both in this country and throughout the world. About 70% of the Americans who've come down with AIDS got the disease from having sex with an infected person.

Most of the teenagers diagnosed with AIDS have also gotten the disease through sexual transmission; however, teenagers account for less than 1% of the U.S. AIDS cases. Because it takes so many years for a person who's infected with the AIDS virus to actually come down with the disease, it's unlikely that teenagers will ever account for a large portion of American AIDS cases. But it's important to remember that 21% of the cases have been people in the 20-to 29-year-old age group. Given the fact that it usually takes several years for an infected person to actually develop a full-blown case of AIDS, we know that many in the 20- to 29-year age group became infected during their teen years.

About 12 million American teenagers have had sexual intercourse. The fact that AIDS is spread mainly through sex and that so many young people are sexually active raises the question of whether the AIDS virus could become widespread among American teens. It's scary to think about the fact that you can get something as deadly as AIDS from something as wonderful as sex. But don't forget: *AIDS can be prevented.* Knowing the facts about sexual transmission will help you understand how to protect yourself against AIDS. So in this chapter we'll be talking about how the virus is passed during sex, what types of sexual activity can spread the disease, and who's at risk of getting AIDS sexually.

How AIDS Is Spread Through Sex

Having some form of sexual intercourse with an infected person is the only sexual activity that has been shown to spread this disease. The AIDS virus can be transmitted during intercourse if viruses from an infected person's body fluids come in contact with the "wet" skin tissues of another person's body. Let me explain exactly what this means.

First of all, as you may recall, the AIDS virus lives in infected people's body fluids. Although the virus can live in a number of different human body fluids, experts believe that only the following fluids actually contain enough viruses to transmit the disease:

- *blood*—this includes menstrual blood, the bloody discharge that females have about once a month, during their menstrual periods
- *semen*—"cum," the mixture of sperm and other sexual fluids released when a male ejaculates
- *vaginal secretions*—various fluids that are produced by glands inside the vagina to keep the skin tissues moist and healthy and to lubricate the vagina during sex
- *possibly, feces*—because feces sometime contain blood
- *possibly, pre-ejaculatory fluid*—the drop or two of fluid that a male may produce from the opening at the tip of his penis when he becomes sexually aroused ("turned on").

It's important to remember that an infected male's pre-ejaculatory fluid may contain AIDS viruses, for this means that it may be possible to get AIDS from having sexual intercourse with an infected male, *even if he doesn't ejaculate or have an orgasm.*[1]

In order to understand how viruses could get from one sex partner's body fluids into the other partner's body during sex, you need to know that human beings have two types of skin tissue, "dry" skin and "wet" skin. "Dry" skin is the kind that covers our arms, legs, face—in fact the entire outside of our bodies. "Wet" skin (whose proper scientific name is *mucous membrane tissue*) is the pink, moist skin tissue that lines the various openings to our bodies—for example, the inside of the mouth, the male urinary opening at the tip if the penis, the inside of the vagina, and the rectum (the lower part of the intestines). The AIDS virus can enter the body through these "wet" skin tissues. In theory, any of these tissues could provide the AIDS virus with a pathway into the body; however, as we shall see, the mouth doesn't appear to be a very likely entry point for the virus.

In Chapter 1, I explained that *the AIDS virus can't infect you unless it gets into your bloodstream.* However, this doesn't mean that you have to have a sore or irritation on your sex organs in order to get AIDS. Scientists believe that the virus may enter the bloodstream during sex in *any* of the following ways:

Open sores, rashes, or irritations in "wet" skin tissue can allow viruses to enter directly into the bloodstream. Sexually transmitted diseases and other infections can cause open sores or rashes that result in breaks in the skin tissues of the sex organs or rectum. Even if there's not a sore, these infections also cause inflammation (irritation, redness, and swelling) of these sensitive tissues. During sex, the inflamed tissues could be rubbed, causing breaks in the skin.

Any bleeding as a result of tearing of the skin tissues during sex could allow the virus to enter the bloodstream. This sort of bleeding is more likely to occur during certain types of intercourse, as we shall see later.

---

[1]When a male ejaculates, he usually has an orgasm, an intense feeling of sexual pleasure. Both males and females experience orgasm, though females don't, of course, ejaculate.

Microscopic breaks in the "wet" skin tissues can also allow the virus to enter the bloodstream. Even when people don't have infections or irritations, there are microscopic breaks (too tiny to be noticed) in the "wet" skin, that is, the mucous membrane tissues of the sex organs. The AIDS virus can infect certain cells of the immune system that travel back and forth between the bloodstream and the tissues just under the mucous membranes. If these cells become infected, they can spread the virus throughout the bloodstream.

It may be possible for the virus to be absorbed directly into the bloodstream through certain cells. There is some evidence to suggest that certain cells in the mucous membrane tissues of the rectum and of the female cervix (the lower part of the uterus, which protrudes into the top of the vagina) can be directly infected by the AIDS virus. If this is so, then infection could occur even if there aren't any microscopic tears or other breaks in the "wet" skin tissues of the rectum or vagina.

The Transmissibility of the AIDS Virus

The AIDS virus is not a highly transmissible virus, i.e., it is not as easily passed from one person to the next as some other germs. Fortunately, the AIDS virus is nowhere near as transmissible as the germs that cause gonorrhea, chlamydia, herpes, syphilis, and some of the other sexually transmitted diseases (STDs). For example, a woman has a 40–50% chance of becoming infected with gonorrhea from just a single act of sexual intercourse with a man who has gonorrhea. But the chances of becoming infected with the AIDS virus after just one act of intercourse with an infected person are nowhere near this high. Although it's true that there have been cases in which men and women have become infected after just one exposure to the AIDS virus, it generally takes *many* repeated exposures for a person to become infected with this virus. In fact, it may take *hundreds* of acts of intercourse with an infected partner before a person becomes infected with the AIDS virus. We'll talk more about the low "infectivity" or "transmissibility" of the AIDS virus later in this chapter, when we discuss the past and future spread of this epidemic.

Factors That Affect a Sex Partner's Chances of Being Infected

One of the big mysteries about AIDS is why some sex partners of infected people have become infected after just one act of intercourse, while others have not yet become infected, despite repeated exposure to the virus. For instance, why do studies of the heterosexual sex partners of infected people show infection rates ranging from a low of zero (no partners infected) to a high of 86%?

Part of the answer is that, as with any germ, some people are just naturally more resistant to the AIDS virus. And some people—those who abuse drugs or alcohol or whose immune systems have been weakened in other ways—are more susceptible to AIDS infection. Other factors that might play a role in determining a person's chances of becoming infected with the AIDS virus as a result of having sex with an infected person are discussed below.

The more often a person is exposed to the virus sexually, the greater the chance of becoming infected. The general rule is: the more often a person has sex with an infected partner or the greater the number of infected partners, the more likely that person is to become infected. (This means that someone who's had lots of sex partners is probably not someone you want as your sex partner.)

The longer the person has been infected, or the more advanced the stage of the disease, the greater the chance that his or her sex partner will also become infected. For instance, it appears that a person who's actually developed symptoms is more likely to infect a sex partner than someone who is still asymptomatic.

Having another sexually transmitted disease increases a person's chance of becoming infected with the AIDS virus. STDs, which are also called *venereal disease* or *VD*, may increase the chances of transmission by causing open sores that would allow the virus direct entry into the bloodstream. Also, when a person has an STD, the immune system sends lots of white blood cells to the area to fight off the STD, and this is the type of cell that the AIDS virus especially likes to infect. Once infected, these cells spread the virus throughout the bloodstream. (For these reasons, it's especially important to have all STDs treated *right away*.)

The type of intercourse that people have may affect their chances of becoming infected. There are three types of intercourse—vaginal, anal, and oral. All three types *may* be capable of spreading the disease, though there is some doubt as to whether oral sex is. And, as we shall see, there's considerable debate over the risk of vaginal vs. anal sex.

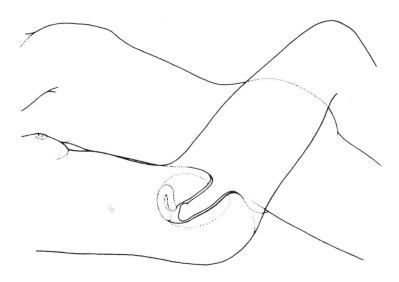

Illustration 3. Vaginal Sex A male or a female can get AIDS from having vaginal intercourse with a sex partner who's infected with the AIDS virus.

Vaginal Sex

Also known as genital sex, this is the most common form of sexual intercourse among heterosexuals. It involves a male putting his penis inside the female vagina (see Illustration 3). Vaginal intercourse is, of course, the way in which human beings reproduce (have babies). If a couple has sex around the time of the month when the female has just produced a ripe ovum (the female egg, or reproductive cell) and a sperm from the male's body joins up with the ovum, pregnancy may result.

During vaginal sex, the "wet" skin that lines the inside of the female's vagina is exposed to her partner's semen. The "wet" skin of the male's urinary opening at the tip of the penis is exposed to her vaginal secretions (including menstrual blood, if they have sex during her period). Thus, *it's possible for a male or a female to get AIDS as a result of having vaginal sex with an infected partner.*

Studies of men and women who've had *short-term* relationships with infected people indicate that it's easier for a male to pass on the AIDS virus to a female than vice versa. There are several reasons why this could be true. For one thing, females have much more "wet" skin exposed during vaginal sex than males. Also, infected semen generally contains a greater number of viruses than infected vaginal secretions. In addition, semen remains in the vagina after sex, but a male is exposed to vaginal secretion only while the couple is actually having sex. However, in studies of men and women in *long-term* relationships, the rates of both male-to-female and female-to-male transmissions are about equal. Generally speaking, roughly half the husbands of women with AIDS, and about half the wives of men with AIDS, become infected.

Oral Sex

Also called *oral-genital sex* or, in slang terms, "69-ing" or "blow jobs," oral sex involves using the mouth or tongue to stimulate another person's sex organs. Both heterosexuals and homosexuals—males as well as females—engage in this form of intercourse. Some couples enjoy oral sex and often include it in their lovemaking. Others have religious or moral objections to it, don't feel comfortable with it, or don't enjoy it, so they don't do it.

Oral sex can be done to either a male or a female. When oral sex is performed on a male, he may ejaculate or he may choose not to do so. If he does ejaculate, his partner may either swallow the semen or spit it out (it has a taste that some people find pleasant, but that others find unpleasant). Even if a female swallows semen, there's no way she could become pregnant, for the semen enters her stomach, and there's no connection between the stomach and the reproductive organs.

Scientists aren't sure if AIDS can be transmitted through oral sex. There is contact between body fluids and "wet" skin during oral sex. For one partner, the contact is between the mouth and either semen or vaginal secretions. For the other, there's contact between the sex organs and his or her partner's saliva (which may contain the AIDS virus—see p. 29). In theory, then, an open sore or other break in the skin of the mouth or sex organs could allow the virus to enter the bloodstream, and because so many viruses are found in infected semen, performing oral sex on a male and swallowing his semen would probably be the riskiest type of oral sex.

However, studies of homosexual men have shown that those who've had only oral sex didn't become infected. Also, in laboratory studies, chimpanzees whose mouths and throats were coated with the virus didn't become infected. On the other hand, there is one study involving the female sex partners of infected men that raises questions about oral sex. In this study, women who had only vaginal sex showed a rate of infection lower than that of women who, in addition to having vaginal sex, also performed oral sex on their male partners. Moreover, there have been reports of at least three cases of AIDS in female homosexuals (lesbians) who claim they've never used IV drugs or had a blood transfusion and whose only possible source of infection seems to be their female partners. If what these women say is true, then it would appear that, at least in some cases, oral sex *can* transmit the disease.

More research is needed, but for now we have to assume

that AIDS can be transmitted through this type of sex, and that therefore oral sex is not totally "safe."

Anal Sex

Also called *rectal intercourse*, this is yet another form of sexual intercourse, and, like oral sex, it can't cause pregnancy. Anal sex involves a male placing his penis into his sex partner's *rectum* (bowels) through the *anus* (the opening through which *feces*, or bowel movements, leave the body).

Some heterosexual couples as well as some male homosexual couples practice anal sex. Some couples enjoy anal sex and often have this form of intercourse. Others don't enjoy it, find it painful, are totally turned off by the whole idea, or disapprove for moral or religious reasons, so they never practice anal sex. As with oral sex, it's a matter of individual choice.

The male who puts his penis into his sex partner's rectum during anal sex is called the *insertive* sex partner (because he *inserts* his penis into the other person). The male or female who *receives* the penis into his or her rectum is called the *receptive* sex partner.

As long as the receptive partner's muscles are relaxed, anal sex usually isn't painful. But if the anal muscles are tense, this type of sex can be uncomfortable or downright painful. There may be some tearing, and possibly bleeding, of the anal or rectal tissues during anal sex, as these tissues are drier and less elastic than, for example, vaginal tissues.

During anal sex the "wet" skin of the receptive sex partner's rectum is exposed to semen. The insertive partner is also at risk because the "wet" skin at the opening of his penis could come in contact with feces left in his partner's rectum or with blood (in cases where there's tearing of the anal or rectal tissues). Thus, it is possible for either a receptive or an insertive partner to get AIDS during anal sex with an infected person.

However, a number of studies have shown that, among homosexuals, the receptive partner is a lot more likely to wind up getting AIDS than the insertive partner. This may be true for a number of reasons, including: a larger number of viruses are found in sperm than in feces; any tearing of the anus or rectal tissues would allow virus in the semen to enter directly into the receptive partner's bloodstream; the rectal mucous membranes may be more susceptible to the virus than those of the male urethra; and the fact that the insertive partner's penis is in contact with the receptive partner's feces or blood only during sex, whereas the semen remains in the receptive partner's rectum for quite a while afterward.

Is Anal Sex Riskier Than Vaginal Sex?

Experts don't yet know whether AIDS is spread more easily through anal sex than through vaginal sex. Most studies of the heterosexual partners of people with AIDS have not shown that heterosexuals who have anal intercourse are more likely to get AIDS than heterosexuals who have only vaginal sex. However, one study of female sex partners of infected men did show that the women who had anal sex were more likely to get AIDS than those who did not. Moreover, this study included larger numbers of women who'd had anal sex than the other studies. Perhaps, as some experts have suggested, larger studies will confirm that anal sex *is* more likely to transmit the disease.

What's important to remember, though, is that *many people have been infected with the AIDS virus by both types of intercourse.* So, please don't think that you're safe from AIDS as long as you don't have anal intercourse.

What About Kissing and French-Kissing?

Because the AIDS virus can live in saliva, some people wonder about the possibility of AIDS being transmitted through kissing. There's no need to worry about getting AIDS from a simple kiss. For one thing, saliva contains only a small number of viruses, and scientists believe that it generally takes a fair amount of the AIDS virus to cause infection. Besides, there's little, if any, saliva exchanged during regular ("dry") kissing.

More saliva may be exchanged during "French-kissing" (putting one's tongue in the other's mouth while kissing). In theory, an open sore or any break in the skin of the mouth or lips could allow viruses in saliva to enter the bloodstream.

But because the amount of virus in saliva is so small, most experts believe there's little, if any, chance of the disease being passed on in this way. Moreover, recent studies suggest that saliva may contain a chemical that helps to inactivate AIDS viruses. Still, scientists can't say it's *absolutely impossible* for AIDS to be transmitted by French-kissing. Therefore, to be on the safe side, you should be careful about who you French-kiss, and you shouldn't do any type of kissing if you have a sore on your lips or in your mouth.

Manual Stimulation (Partner Masturbation) Is "Safe"

Manual stimulation is also called partner masturbation. *Manual* means "by hand." *Masturbation* means touching, rubbing, or stroking the sex organs, and it's something people may do by themselves in private, with someone else, or to someone else.

The AIDS virus cannot pass through unbroken "dry" skin. As long as you don't have a cut or break in the skin of your hands, there is no danger of getting AIDS from manual stimulation. Even if you had a cut on your hand and got someone's semen or vaginal secretions in the cut, it is unlikely that you'd get AIDS. (If, however, the cut is infected, this increases your chances of getting AIDS, see pages 86–87). To be on the safe side, though, you should not masturbate someone else if you have a cut on your hand, regardless of whether or not it's infected.

Now that you know the basic facts about sexual transmission, let's talk about the sexual spread of the AIDS epidemic among American heterosexuals.

Will AIDS Become Widespread Among American Heterosexuals?

There's now no doubt that AIDS will become widespread among American heterosexuals who belong to certain risk groups, namely IV drug users and their sex partners. But what about heterosexuals who don't belong to these or any of the other risk groups? Will there be significant spread beyond the risk groups, and into the general heterosexual population? Or will the epidemic continue to be confined mostly to Americans who are homosexual/bisexual males, IV drug abusers, hemophiliac/transfusion recipients, and the sex partners of people in these risk groups?

As I explained in Chapter 1, we don't yet have the complete answer to this question. But in the following pages, we'll be taking a look at what *is* known. Unfortunately, news reports on TV or in the papers often make it sound as if this question has been answered one way or the other. As a result, the American public has gone from thinking that there's absolutely no chance of AIDS becoming widespread among heterosexuals, to being convinced that a heterosexual epidemic of major proportions was just around the corner, and then back to thinking that heterosexuals are safe from AIDS. As we shall see, *none* of these things are true.

The AIDS Epidemic Among Gay Men

One common misconception is that the reason why so many male homosexuals and bisexuals in this country are infected is that anal sex is an especially effective way of transmitting the AIDS virus. Of course, the flip side of this theory is that vaginal sex is much less likely to transmit the disease and, therefore, AIDS will never become widespread among U.S. heterosexuals. However, as I explained in the last section, it's not entirely clear that anal sex is a "better" way of spreading the disease. And, even if it is, vaginal sex is *also* an effective way of spreading the virus. For instance, in one recent study, there was an 86% infection rate among women who continued having vaginal sex with their husbands in the first year after the men were diagnosed as having AIDS.

Moreover, 90% of the women with AIDS interviewed in the United States, Africa, and Europe said they'd never had anal sex. (Many of them didn't even know what anal sex *was*!) And in Africa, where anal sex is rarely practiced, virtually all sexual transmission takes place between heterosexuals, through vaginal sex. Since the epidemic is more widespread there than anywhere else, it's clearly possible to create and sustain a widespread epidemic through vaginal sex alone.

What many people don't realize is that *it's not so much the kind of intercourse, but the performing of sex with a large number of individual partners which accounts for the AIDS epidemic in homosexual and bisexual males.* Before AIDS was recognized, many gay men had large numbers of sex partners. For instance, in a 1978 study of 685 gay men, about 72% reported having had 100 or more different partners; 27% had had *1000* or more. Consider what this meant in terms of AIDS. Say, for example, that an infected homosexual had 100 different sex partners before he even realized he had AIDS. If he infected 1 out of every 10 of his 100 partners, he infected 10 men. If each of these men also had 100 partners and infected 10 of them, there'd be a total of 100 newly infected men. If each of those men infected 10 there'd be 1000, then 10,000, and so on. Once the disease became this widespread, even gay men who had only two or three sex partners had a fairly high risk of becoming infected. Unfortunately, because of the fact that it takes so many years for the symptoms to develop, AIDS infection was already widespread before anybody even realized what was going on.

As you can see, having a large number of sexual partners (sometimes termed *casual sex* or *promiscuity*) can quickly create an epidemic, and that's exactly what happened in the gay community—there was an *explosive* growth of cases among homosexual and bisexual men. As you'll learn in Chapter 4, the same sort of mathematics accounts for the wide and rapid spread of AIDS among IV drug users in the "shooting galleries" of New York and other major urban areas in the northeast. Moreover, large numbers of sex partners is also the major factor in the African AIDS epidemic.

The Heterosexual Epidemic in Africa

In 1986 an increasing number of stories about AIDS in Africa began to appear in the American news media. These stories revealed that the number of AIDS cases was growing at an even more explosive rate in Africa than in the U.S. As in the U.S., the disease was being transmitted primarily through sex, but in Africa, the virus was being spread by *heterosexuals* through *vaginal sex.* As a result of these reports America suddenly decided that far from being "safe" from AIDS, U.S. heterosexuals were about to experience an outbreak of AIDS cases that would make the Black Plague (which wiped out more than one-third of the population of Europe in the 1300s) "pale by comparison."

The fact of the matter is that there are important differences between African and American heterosexuals, including:

- The average African isn't as healthy as the average American. Because their immune system may be weaker to begin with, Africans could be more susceptible to AIDS.
- Sterile needles aren't always available to African doctors and hospitals. So some African heterosexuals have become infected through dirty IV needles. (This doesn't account for the spread of AIDS in rural Africa where *no* healthcare is available.)
- Sexually transmitted diseases (STDs) are more common in Africa and, due to lack of healthcare, may go untreated.

But perhaps the key factor in the AIDS epidemic in Africa is the role of prostitutes. Prostitution is much more common in Africa than it is in the U.S. For instance, at truck stops along the major highway in Central Africa (a route that goes through the area where many scientists believe that the AIDS virus originated), prostitutes wait at roadside shacks, available for hire to any trucker who happens to stop. And many prostitutes in Africa, like many homosexual men in the U.S., have an unusually large number of sex partners, more than 1000 partners in some studies. *Just as with American homosexuals, it is the large numbers of sex partners that is the major cause of the wide and rapid spread of AIDS in Africa.*

The Sexual Spread of AIDS Among U.S. Heterosexuals

AIDS is spreading among the female sex partners of male IV drug users, but experts disagree sharply over the question of whether AIDS will ever become widespread among

American heterosexuals who don't belong to an AIDS risk group.

Most experts don't think we'll ever see the kind of explosive growth of AIDS cases among American heterosexuals that there's been among American gays and African heterosexuals. The AIDS virus is not highly transmissible, so explosive growth requires large numbers of sex partners. But very few American heterosexuals have as many partners as American gay men and African prostitutes. It's true that the infection rate among prostitutes in some U.S. cities is high. But prostitution is less widespread in this country, and, unlike prostitutes in Africa, here they often use condoms, which helps prevent the spread of AIDS.

Because they feel that U.S. prostitutes are not likely to be a major factor in the spreading of AIDS, and because other heterosexuals in the U.S. don't usually have large numbers of sex partners, most experts don't expect an explosive growth of AIDS cases in the general heterosexual population. It is important to remember, though, that no cure or vaccine for AIDS is expected in the near future, if ever, and there is considerable disagreement over the question of what will happen in the long run. Right now, even by the CDC's estimates (which many consider too low), there are over a quarter of a million infected heterosexuals in the U.S. Many experts believe that this is enough to eventually sustain a widespread heterosexual epidemic in the U.S.

The truth is that no one can tell right now how common AIDS will become among heterosexuals in this country. Even experts who are convinced that there won't be an explosive growth of cases among heterosexuals outside the risk groups say that no one really knows that will happen in the years to come.

Take, for example, Dr. Harold Jaffee, who's the chief epidemiologist in the CDC's AIDS program and one of the experts who thinks it's *very* unlikely that there will be an explosive growth. Dr. Jaffee was quoted in the March 14, 1988, issue of *People* magazine:

> Those who are suggesting that we are going to see an explosive spread of AIDS in the heterosexual population have to explain why this isn't happening.

Yet, in the same article, Dr. Jaffee also said:

> Over the next 5, 10, 15, 20 years? I don't think anybody knows . . . Will there be sustained transmission into the general population? Some people have predicted that it won't happen, others predict it's inevitable. I don't think we know.

Another thing you need to remember is that, regardless of whether or not AIDS spreads widely into the general heterosexual population, *all experts agree that there will be some spread of AIDS among heterosexuals that don't belong to a risk group.* In fact, there already has been. Since heterosexual transmission can and does happen, *all sexually active people must learn how to protect themselves from this disease.*

Teenagers, Sex, and AIDS

As I pointed out at the beginning of this chapter, because it takes several years for an infected person to actually come down with AIDS, it's unlikely that teenagers will ever account for a large portion of the *full-blown* cases of AIDS. But if this epidemic does spread into the general population, *infection* with the AIDS virus may become very widespread among teens. After all, AIDS is basically a sexually transmitted disease and millions of today's teenagers are having sex. The following things all increase the risk of AIDS: IV drug use, homosexuality, prostitution, sexually transmitted diseases, a high level of sexual activity, and multiple partners. If you'll look at the chart in Illustration 4, you'll see that as a group, American teenagers have all these risk factors.

Even if you aren't in a risk group and don't have a risk factor, please remember: *If you're having sex, you may be at risk for AIDS.*

You Can Be In a Risk Group Without Knowing It

There are more than a few people in this country who had no idea that they were the sex partners of people in risk groups until they developed AIDS. Neither IV drug users nor the people in the other risk groups have neon signs on

SEXUAL ACTIVITY
An estimated 11.5 million teenagers between the ages of 13 and 19 have had sexual intercourse.

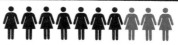

5 million females
7 of every 10 by age 20

6.5 million males
8 of every 10 by age 20

MULTIPLE PARTNERS
Many teens have had a large number of different sex partners.

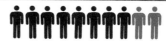

1 of every 6 teen women have had four or more partners

MALE HOMOSEXUAL ACTIVITY
In one survey, 17% of male teenagers reported having had at least one homosexual experience; 2% were currently having sex with other males.

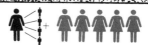

1 of every 6 teen men has had one or more homosexual experiences

SEXUALLY TRANSMITTED DISEASES
Each year, 2.5 million teenagers contract gonorrhea, herpes, syphilis, or one of the other STDs.

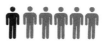

1 of every 6 teenagers develops an STD

PROSTITUTION
An estimated 125,000 to 200,000 teenage men and women become involved in prostitution each year. About 2/3 of these teens are runaways; 1/3 live with their parents or guardians.

IV DRUG USE
In a 1986 study of high school seniors, 1.1% had used heroin within the past year and 13% had taken cocaine, some by needle. Experts estimate that at least 200,000 teens have used IV drugs.

Illustration 4. American Teens and AIDS Risk

their foreheads. And it's not just a certain "type" of person who's bisexual or who uses IV drugs, as two female college students recently learned. Both of these coeds had sex with the same white, middle-class male student at a major university. Although he didn't seem the "type," this male student was an IV drug user, a fact which neither of these girls discovered until they'd been infected with the AIDS virus. Please remember that if you're having sex you can get AIDS even if you don't think you're in one of the risk groups and don't have one of the risk factors in Illustration 4.

Your Partner's Past Sex Partners Can Pose a Threat to You

When you have sex with someone nowadays, in a sense you're not just having sex with that person, but also with everyone that person's ever had sex with. Let me give you an example of what I mean. Take Charles, for instance. As his girlfriend, Jackie, explained to me:

> Charles thinks there's no way he could ever get AIDS. He thinks it's just impossible because he's just so macho. He thinks he's invincible.

Charles is wrong. What Charles doesn't realize is that one of Jackie's ex-boyfriends occasionally used IV drugs, and when he did, he shared needles. Moreover, Jackie's ex-boyfriend was also at risk for AIDS because he sometimes had sex with other males.

Jackie and her ex-boyfriend had sex frequently, so if he was infected—either from sharing needles or from having sex with other males—then he may well have passed the virus on to her. If so, Jackie could, in turn, pass it on to Charles. So as I said, Charles is wrong. There *is* a way he could get AIDS.

Don't make the same mistake as Charles. Unless you know *all* your sex partners *very* well and you *also* know about *all* their past sex partners, you just can't say there's "no way" you could get AIDS.

Think in Terms of "Risky Behaviors," Not "Risk Groups"

Thinking in terms of "risk groups" instead of "risky behaviors" can be very dangerous. Let me give you an example. Joe and Sue (not their real names), students at a college in a southern state, had a sexual relationship. Joe had never used IV drugs or had a blood transfusion. Except for two sexual experiences with a male friend, all his sexual partners had been females. So Joe didn't consider himself a homosexual or bisexual, and he wasn't an IV drug user or transfusion recipient. And he thought he wasn't in a risk group. But Joe did engage in *risky behavior* when he had sex with his male friend. As it turned out, Joe became infected from having sex with his male friend, and Sue is now infected with the AIDS virus as well.

So, please remember, it's *what you do* that puts you at risk for AIDS, *not who you "are."*

The Good News (Yes, There Is Some Good News)

Believe it or not, there actually *is* some good news regarding AIDS and teens:

Experts believe that right now, the infection rate among teenagers is quite low. Although AIDS infection among teenagers is on the rise and is very high among the female sex partners of male IV drug users, experts believe that the infection rate in the general teenage population is quite low.

You can keep it that way. AIDS can be stopped! In Chapter 3, you'll learn what you need to do to help prevent the sexual spread of this disease. I know you wouldn't want to harm others or yourself. So learn what needs to be done and do it!

Please remember, the decisions your generation makes about sex and drugs may well determine the future course of this epidemic. If it turns out that AIDS *is* capable of spreading into the general population, your generation may turn out to be the most important generation to ever walk the face of this planet. In fact, if AIDS is capable of spreading as widely as some fear, what this generation of young people does or doesn't do in terms of sex and drugs may determine the future course of human civilization! The human race has a lot riding on you . . . Carry it well.

CHAPTER THREE

Preventing Sexual Transmission:
Abstinence and Safer Sex

I HATE HAVING to warn the teenagers in my classes about the dangers of AIDS and tell them, "Be careful, or you'll get this deadly disease." I hate it that my 18-year-old daughter and you and all the other young people of this generation have to contend with this nightmare of a disease that has linked love and sex with death. But my hating it doesn't change the facts, and one of those facts is:

> TEENAGERS MUST EITHER ABSTAIN FROM (NOT HAVE) SEX OR, IF THEY DO HAVE SEX, THEY MUST TAKE STEPS TO HELP PROTECT THEMSELVES AGAINST AIDS.

Notice, I didn't say "some" teenagers. I didn't say "certain" teenagers or "high risk" teenagers. *All* teenagers—unless they are abstaining from sex—need to take precautions to reduce the risk of getting AIDS. Taking these precautions is called practicing "safer sex" and involves following three guidelines: 1) Limit the number of sex partners you have; 2) Choose your sex partners carefully; and 3) Use a latex condom ("rubber") each and every time you have sex. In this chapter, I'll be explaining these guidelines and how to make sure that you and your sexual partners follow them.

Practicing safer sex will greatly reduce your risk of getting AIDS. In fact, as long as you follow *all three* guidelines correctly and consistently, there's very little chance of your getting AIDS. However, you should be aware that *practicing safer sex doesn't absolutely guarantee that you'll be safe from AIDS*. Remember: even if you limit yourself to only one partner, if that one partner happened to be infected, you could get AIDS too. And no matter how careful you are about choosing partners, it's still possible to have sex with an infected person. Moreover, even if you use condoms each and every time you have sex, the fact is condoms are just not 100% effective in preventing transmission of the AIDS virus. So although practicing safer sex *reduces* the risk of getting AIDS, it does not *eliminate* the risk.

The only way to completely eliminate the risk of sexual transmission of AIDS is to abstain from sexual intercourse. In the first section of this chapter, then, we'll be talking about abstaining from sex until you're married or at least until you've finished your teen years and are an adult. We'll also be talking about how you can be sexually intimate and even have orgasms without any risk of AIDS. Of course, AIDS isn't the only reason or even the main one for teens to abstain from sexual intercourse. But even if you wouldn't otherwise abstain, you should be aware of the fact that it makes particularly good sense to abstain for at least the coming year or so. By then, the results of some important AIDS studies will be in, and we'll have a much clearer idea of how widespread the disease is and just how much risk there is in having sex.

Abstinence

Why Wait? Some Reasons for Abstaining
Other than AIDS, why wait to have sex? Different people have different answers to this question. Dr. Sol Gordon,

the famous sex educator, tells why he thinks teenagers should not have sex[1]:

> . . . Even committed relationships are spoiled by premature and early sex. Boys think they know everything, girls think that boys can teach them everything—it doesn't work that way. The first experience of sex is usually pretty grim. Almost no girl will have an orgasm. The boy gets his orgasm three days later when he tells the guys about it . . . People think that if you *really* love each other you're going to have this great experience— you know, bells will ring, firecrackers will sound. It doesn't happen that way. It sometimes takes months and years before people really get to know each other sexually.

Another man explains why he's glad that he waited until he was married to have sex:

> Learning about sex together, with each other, made it that much more special . . . We really trusted each other, and that made us feel safe enough for us to really "let go." We didn't have to worry that if we did it "wrong" or it wasn't great the first time that it would all be over. If we hadn't been married and hadn't already promised to be there through thick and thin with each other, I think it would have been harder to learn to have good sex.

A teenager girl tells about her reasons for abstaining:

> I have girlfriends who think if you get into heavy petting and all with a boy, it's stupid or artificial or something not to go all the way and have sex with him. They say sex isn't such a big deal . . . Maybe I'm too romantic or too idealistic, but I think sex is a big deal, or should be. I want it to be very deep and very emotional . . . I know you can go around having sex all the time and it won't be a big deal for you. If you do that too much, though, I think you get . . . well, hard and cold and kind of callous.

Many teens choose to abstain because premarital sex goes against their religious or moral beliefs. Many choose to

---

[1]Quoted from Dr. Gordon's video *Sex: A Topic for Conversation for Teenagers*—a terrific video. You can order it from Mondell Productions, Inc., 5215 Homer Street, Dallas, Texas 75206 (214) 826-3863.

wait because they just don't feel they're "ready" yet, or they sense that their relationships need time to grow first. Then, too, there's the possibility of pregnancy and the question of whether you're ready to handle having to choose between adoption, abortion, and parenthood. Sexually transmitted diseases (STDs) are another consideration, for they can cause serious health problems, especially for women, who may lose their ability to ever have children because of an STD.

If you're not sure how you feel about abstinence, why not talk this over with someone older whom you trust? After all, it's an important decision; why not get the benefit of someone else's experience? (Don't, as many young people do, automatically rule out your parents as people to talk to. You may be surprised to find that they struggled with the same issue when they were your age!)

Sticking to Your Decision

If you choose to abstain, the following advice can help you stick to your decision:

Discuss your decision with your boyfriend or girlfriend. If it turns out that you both feel the same way, great! If not, then being clear right from the beginning may help the other person understand that it's not a reflection of your feelings for him or her, and he or she will be less likely to feel hurt or rejected.

Don't set yourself up. Drinking, using drugs, being alone together when your parents won't be home for hours— these sorts of things are "set-ups," situations that will *not* help you stick to your decision. So, use your common sense and don't set yourself up.

Be aware of the fact that there's a great deal of social and peer pressure to have sex. Sex is everywhere in our society. Rock lyrics tell us to, "Do it, do it, do it!"; TV ads use sex to sell toothpaste. Movies make it seem as if *all* teenagers are having sex, and the papers are full of statistics like, "Half of America's teenagers are having sex!" But remember: if half of American teenagers are having sex, that also means that half aren't; the media doesn't give a *real* picture of teen life; and the rock singer won't send you a get well card if you get AIDS.

Peer pressure may take many different forms. It may be other people your age acting as if there's something "wrong" with you or implying that you're neurotic or homosexual if you don't want to have sex. Friends who've had sex may take the attitude that they're mature, terribly sophisticated, and totally hip, while you, poor thing, are still a mere child. Or, if you admit to being a virgin, they may say, "What! You're *still* a virgin???" And, of course, the way they say it makes it sound like you just confessed that you still wear diapers or have some hideously vile habit like eating toads for breakfast.

Don't let this sort of thing get to you! Forget peer pressure and go with your own thoughts, feelings, and values.

Don't let a boyfriend or girlfriend pressure you into sex. Supposedly guys are the ones who do the pressuring, but I get plenty of letters from male readers who say it's their girlfriends who are pressuring them. Either way, pressuring is just not OK!

Don't let anyone con you into having sex to "prove" your love; sex is never a test of love. And if someone tries to blackmail you by saying, "If you won't have sex, I'll leave you," wave goodbye! I absolutely guarantee you that this person *will* leave you sooner or later, regardless of whether or not you agree to have sex. Don't fall for a "line." If someone hands you a line, hand them one right back:

IF HE/SHE SAYS:	YOU CAN SAY:
Everyone else is doing it.	Good, then you shouldn't have much trouble finding someone to do it with.
Prove you love me by having sex with me.	Prove you love me by not pressuring me.
What's the matter, don't you want me?	Yes, and I want what's right for both of us.

IF HE/SHE SAYS:	YOU CAN SAY:
It's not such a big deal.	Then I *definitely* don't want to do it.
Half the guys/girls I know would give their right arm for a chance to go to bed with me.	So start a right arm collection.

Remember, if sex "just happens," you might "just happen" to get AIDS. Teens often say that they weren't really planning to have sex, it "just happened." Regardless of whether or not you choose to abstain, it's important that you *consciously* think through the whole issue so that it's part of your awareness. That way, there's less chance that sex will "just happen" to you. Remember, too, that intercourse isn't the only way of being sexual.

Outercourse: A Safe, Satisfying Way of Being Intimate

Sharing a good sexual experience can bring a rush of good feelings, a sense of intimacy, a special closeness between two people. Sexual intercourse is just about as close as two people can get. Unfortunately, for many teens, intercourse is not a wonderful experience. Often the boy becomes excited and has an orgasm right away, and the girl doesn't have one at all. He feels inadequate because he "came" so fast; she feels inadequate because she didn't "come" at all. Instead of closeness and intimacy, there's distance; instead of fireworks, there's fizzle (or worse).

Before I ever did it, it was like, "Oh, wow, sex!", like doing it with a girl was going to be the best thing ever. But, when we did it, it was, "Oh, well, that was nice."

It was just this boy on top of me. It was nothing. It didn't hurt too much, but it wasn't special. It wasn't nice . . . Really, I hated it. It was nothing.

Safe sex activities (or "outercourse" as I call them in my class) are ways of expressing affection and love, of being close, and of sharing physical pleasure and intimacy without the risk of AIDS. Any activity that is "dry," that doesn't involve the exchange of body fluids, is safe because there's no risk of getting AIDS. As long as there's no contact between "wet" skin and body fluids, all of the following activities are safe:

- Dry kissing, (not "wet" or French-kissing, though[2])
- Hugging
- Body-to-body rubbing
- Massage/Petting
- Manual stimulation[3]
- Partner masturbation[3]

You may have moral objections to some of these things. Or you may not feel comfortable with or interested in or ready for some of these activities. Just because they're safe from the point of view of AIDS doesn't mean they're right for you. You never have to do anything you don't want to do, no matter how safe it is!

Deciding "how far" you want to go isn't always easy. Reading books like this one or talking to your parents, boyfriend or girlfriend, other friends your own age, or older friends can help you decide. Sometimes, though, you may not know until afterward that something wasn't "right" for you. For instance, you may experiment with heavy petting (touching each other's sex organs or a girl's breasts under her clothes) and feel bad about it later. But that's how we learn—by our mistakes—and if you don't feel good about something you've done, you can always decide not to do it again.

If you've been having intercourse or are considering doing so, I hope you'll consider outercourse, as an alternative to intercourse. Outercourse can be a way of changing

---

[2]French-kissing may not be safe. If you've forgotten why, see pages 29–30.
[3]This is safe as long as there is no broken skin (see page 30). Also, see page 30, if you've forgotten what these terms mean.

your sex life for the better. Instead of the penis in the vagina as in intercourse, you can use safe-sex activities like body-to-body rubbing, massage, manual stimulation, and partner masturbation to express sexual feelings and also to achieve orgasm. This means, first of all, that females are more likely to have an orgasm. In case you don't know, 75% of women do not have an orgasm from the penis moving in and out of the vagina, but require manual stimulation. Secondly, it means that you and your partner are more likely to *communicate* about what feels good to each of you sexually. Despite what we're led to believe from books and movies, great lovers don't automatically know how to please their partners sexually. But they do know how to communicate and find out what feels good to that particular person.

Last but not least, outercourse can bring the intimacy that is so often lacking in teenagers' sexual experience. As the well-known sex therapist Dr. Helen Singer Kaplan has said, "By observing each other's arousal and climax [orgasm], you are sharing a very private experience with each other. You are allowing yourselves to be vulnerable with each other . . . when two people let their guards down, and see that they will not get hurt, it makes them feel more loving and close to each other."

Having outercourse may mean overcoming shyness. It may involve much more intimacy than you've ever had from intercourse, and that can be scary. But if you've been having sex, yet don't feel you could possibly have outercourse, perhaps you're not ready for the emotional intensity of a sexual relationship at all. If so, do yourself a favor and wait until you are ready.

If you and your partner do decide to try outercourse, the urge to have intercourse may be very strong. However, by satisfying yourselves in these other ways, you'll be able to "hold out." Remember, though, the exchange of body fluids can spread AIDS, so make sure there's no contact between body fluids and "wet" skin.

If you should decide to have sex, make sure that you first understand and follow all three of the safer-sex guidelines below.

Practicing Safer Sex

In this section, you'll find lots of practical advice to help you and your partner talk about safer sex and follow the three guidelines. I hope I haven't made it sound as if practicing safer sex is as easy as one, two, three—because it's not. For one thing, there's all this business about "real men" (who, of course, never turn down a chance to have sex) and "nice girls" (who aren't looking to have sex). A "real man" is going to have problems choosing sex partners carefully, and "nice girls" are hardly supposed to go to the store and buy condoms!

For another thing, there's all the goofy, unrealistic ideas about sex that television has been programming into our brains ever since we were little kids. According to one research group, a typical American kid sees more than 9,000 "situations implying sexual intercourse" in the course of a single year's TV viewing! But TV "teaches" us that a) sex rarely has negative consequences and b) people never discuss things like preventing disease or pregnancy before having sex. Think about it—do characters on soap operas get gonorrhea? Does anyone on "Dynasty" get herpes? How often do you hear characters on TV say anything like, "Excuse me, but do you have a condom?" or "Before we have sex, shouldn't we talk about birth control and about protecting ourselves against sexually transmitted diseases, especially AIDS?"

The fact is, in TV-land, where sex is always glamorous and trouble-free, people rarely *talk* about having sex at all, they just do it. But if you're going to practice safer sex, you have to understand that there can indeed be negative consequences to having sex and that you have to discuss these things beforehand.

It *is* possible, though, to take charge of your own sex life and make it a safer one. I know, because I know teens who are doing it. So, hang in there, get tough, and get safe!

Talking to a Potential Sex Partner About Safer Sex

Telling someone that you plan to use condoms or questioning potential sex partners about their past sex lives (not to mention having to talk about your own) can be really embarrassing and awkward. Remember, though, that unlike AIDS, embarrassment doesn't last for the rest of your life and you don't die from it. Besides, once you've managed to get past the initial stages, embarrassment fades pretty quickly.

As you'll learn later in this chapter, you'll need to discuss all sorts of things with your partner before you'll be ready to make love. And this isn't the sort of thing you can take care of in one five- or ten-minute conversation. In fact, the two of you will have to do *lots* of talking and have many, many conversations before you're ready for sex.

You might want to start out by talking about AIDS and safer sex in a general way—the same way you'd discuss any other current event or news story. Or perhaps you'll want to jump right into talking about safer sex in a more personal way, in terms of your relationship with each other. However you go about it, the following tips can help make things go more smoothly.

First, learn everything you can about AIDS and safer sex. If you have the facts straight in your own mind, you'll feel more confident and do a better job of communicating.

Plan what you want to say and how to say it. This will also help you to feel more comfortable and more confident. Since getting started can be the hardest part, you might want to rehearse some "opening lines":

> I've been hearing all this stuff about AIDS and it's got me pretty scared. How do you feel about the whole AIDS thing?
>
> I have a lot of friends who are having sex, but who aren't doing anything to protect themselves from AIDS. I don't see taking chances, not with something as deadly as AIDS. What about you? What do you think people ought to do about AIDS?
>
> I feel embarrassed talking about this and it's hard for me to even bring the subject up. But I think we need to talk about AIDS and safer sex.

> Look, I'm not interested in having babies and I'll bet you're not, either. And, for sure, we don't want to get AIDS, so let's talk about how we're going to protect ourselves.

Keep your sense of humor and if you're embarrassed, say so. AIDS is serious business. But it's OK to laugh and joke, and it's also OK to be embarrassed. You don't have to pretend you're Mr. and Ms. Totally Cool. Admitting you're nervous or embarrassed takes the pressure off both of you.

Listen to what your partner has to say and pay attention to his or her reaction. Does your partner have a lot of mistaken ideas about AIDS? If so, you'll need to spend some time explaining what you've learned about AIDS. You might read all or part of this book together.

Be aware of the fact that the other person may react negatively. He or she may be relieved and grateful that you've brought the topic up, but some people do get turned off or feel insulted and may even put you down for wanting to talk about protecting yourself from AIDS. The following "lines" will help to make you aware of, and to deal with, some of these negative reactions:

IF HE/SHE SAYS:	YOU COULD SAY:
Don't tell me you're one of those nuts who's all in a panic about AIDS!	I'm not in a panic, but I am concerned. After all, this isn't measles we're talking about. Or: Yep, I am one of those nuts.
The media is just making a mountain out of a molehill. People like us don't have to worry about getting AIDS.	The media does use scare tactics, but I think there's a real reason for concern. Even the experts disagree. Until they figure it out, I'm playing it safe.

IF HE/SHE SAYS:	YOU CAN SAY:
I didn't think you were the type that needed to be concerned about AIDS. Now I'm beginning to wonder.	Everybody needs to be concerned, not just certain "types" of people. After all, AIDS can infect anyone.
I'm a virgin, there's no way I could have AIDS.	I'm not. By practicing safer sex, we'll both be protected.
I know I'm clean. I haven't had sex with anyone in months.	Thanks, I really appreciate your honesty. As far as I know, I'm not infected either. But just in case we're wrong, let's protect ourselves.
I love you. I wouldn't give you AIDS.	Not on purpose, but people can be infected without even realizing it.
What an insult! Do you think I have AIDS? Do you think I'm gay? Or: I'm not that kind of girl!	I didn't mean to insult you and if I thought you had AIDS, I wouldn't even *consider* sleeping with you. But the fact is, nowadays, just about anyone can be infected.

Now that you've got a general idea of how to talk about AIDS and safer sex, let's look at what's involved in actually practicing safer sex.

Safer Sex Guideline #1: Limit the Number of Sex Partners You Have

Let's face it: the freewheeling days of the 60s and 70s are over. AIDS has changed all that. Casual sex—having sex on a "casual" basis or with people you only know casually—is just too dangerous these days. For one thing, you'll wind up having far too many sex partners that way. With AIDS, there's safety in numbers ... *low* numbers, that is. The fewer partners you have, the lower your risk.

To limit the number of sex partners you have, take your

time and get to know a person well before you have sex. It's also important to only have sex when it's a monogamous relationship, that is, one where you're committed to only having sex with each other. After all, if your partner is having sex with other people, he or she could bring the virus home to you. So, before you have sex, talk about the fact that you're expecting a one-on-one relationship. You don't want to find out later that your partner had a "no-strings-attached" relationship in mind. And make a mutual promise to tell right away if you aren't faithful. Making this promise is no guarantee, but it does increase the chances of honesty if either of you is unfaithful.

To keep the number of sex partners you have to a minimum:

Don't sleep with someone you've just met or hardly know and don't make spur-of-the-moment decisions. Even with someone you know well, don't make the decision to have sex hastily. As one girl put it:

> You can't be spontaneous. You can't be loose. Those things just can't happen anymore. You've got to give it careful consideration. You can't act on impulse.

Slow down! Don't be in a rush to include intercourse in your relationship. Intercourse doesn't have to be a part of a relationship right away—or ever, for that matter. Give the relationship some time to develop. It's OK to wait months, years even, before you start having sex with each other. And remember: intercourse isn't the only way to have orgasms. You can be sexual with someone without the risk of AIDS or pregnancy by having outercourse (pages 45–47).

Before you decide to have sex, ask yourself if you honestly think the two of you will be together a year from now. You don't have a crystal ball, and you can't give a definite answer. However, if (in all honesty) you doubt the relationship will last a year, then you ought to forgo sex. By having short-term relationships, you can end up with far too many sex partners.

The fact that you're not a virgin doesn't mean you have to include sex in every relationship. A new relationship may be just as intense or long-lasting as a past relationship that included sex, but that doesn't necessarily mean you have to have sex with your new partner. If you're being pressured to have sex to "prove" you love your new partner just as much as a former partner, explain that your decision doesn't have anything to do with love—just safety.

Be very careful if someone has just ended a sexual relationship with you. It hurts to be rejected and it's easy to get involved in a new sexual relationship "on the rebound." A new love is a great cure for a broken heart, but don't rush into having sex with a new partner as a "cure" for rejection.

Safer Sex Guideline #2:
Choose Your Sex Partners Carefully

> My dad told me, "Find out everything. Really find out *everything* about a person" . . . if they did drugs, what kind of people they've had sex with before . . . maybe they had a transfusion when they were just a little kid or something.
>
> I'm real up-front with it. I say, "Here's the people I've had sex with," and tell them about my past sex life. I expect them to tell me the same. If he doesn't want to say, hems or haws, or makes sounds like he's leaving . . . Goodby!

The idea behind this guideline is, of course, to avoid having sex with someone who's infected with the AIDS virus. After all, if the condom breaks or comes off during sex (which happens) and your partner is infected, you could get AIDS. Therefore, you want to choose your partners *very* carefully.

One thing you need to remember here is that it can take years for AIDS symptoms to show up and most of the 1.5 million Americans who are carrying the AIDS virus don't even know that they're infected. So, you can't choose safe sex partners just by looking for symptoms or asking, "Do you have AIDS? Are you infected?" Instead, you need to find out whether a person has done things which are likely to have exposed him or her to the AIDS virus—for example, using IV drugs, having sex with drug users, having sex with a male homosexual or male bisexual. Obviously, someone you've just met or hardly know isn't going to share this kind of information with you. ("Not if they're after your bod," as one girl put it.) In order for this guideline to work, you have to take the time to develop a strong mutual trust and a truly caring relationship *before* you have sex. People who are at-risk for AIDS aren't going to tell you about this unless they know you *very* well and have come to trust and care for you. There are some people who'll be dishonest no matter how well they know you or care for you. But if they're given enough time (and are approached in the right way) the majority of people will volunteer this sort of information rather than risk infecting someone they care about.

AIDS Antibody Testing Is No Substitute for Knowing Your Partner Well

If your partner is at-risk for AIDS, it may be necessary to have AIDS antibody testing or to simply not have intercourse with this person. But while antibody testing can play an important role in choosing safe partners, testing is only useful if you know a person *very* well and feel very sure that he/she has abstained from sex and drugs for at least the entire six months directly prior to the test and will continue to abstain from IV drugs or from having sex with anyone other than you. (Remember, a person can test negative one day, and the next day go out and have sex or share needles and become infected. And it can take as long as six months for a person to develop enough antibodies to show up on the test.) So it's very important that you know the person very well—well enough to trust that the things this person tells you about him or herself are true.

AIDS Risk Factors

A person is at-risk for getting or spreading the AIDS virus if the person:

1. has AIDS or ARC or has tested positive for the AIDS antibody or has had sex with such a person.[4]
2. has ever used needles to take illegal drugs or has had sex with such a person.
3. is a male who has had sex with another male even once since 1977[5] or is a female who has had sex with a bisexual male.
4. has hemophilia or another clotting disorder and has received clotting factor concentrates[6] at any time between 1977 and the spring of 1985 or has had sex with such a person.
5. has lived in or traveled to Africa or to Haiti at any time since 1977 and received a needle injection from a doctor or anyone else while in that country or had sexual intercourse while there.
6. has been a male or female prostitute at any time since 1977 or has had sex with such a person.
7. received a blood transfusion between 1977 and the spring of 1985.
8. has had gonorrhea, chlamydia, herpes, syphilis or another sexually transmitted disease.
9. has had sex with a number of different partners.

---

[4]Whether knowingly or not.
[5]The AIDS virus had undoubtedly been around since before 1977, but that's the first year when it had spread widely enough to be of any real concern. Thus, the year 1977 is used throughout this list.
[6]If you've forgotten what a hemophiliac is or want to know about clotting factor concentrates, see pages 81–82.

How to Talk to a Potential Partner About Risk Factors

You might begin by saying something like:

> We need to talk about possible risk of infection. What's happened in my life, what's happened in your life that could have possibly exposed either of us to the virus?

Or, you might say:

> I really care for you and I want us both to be safe, so let's talk about AIDS antibody testing. Do we need to consider testing before we go ahead and make love?

You could also begin by volunteering your own sexual history—saying how many sex partners you've had, who your past partners have been, and so forth. This opens the door and encourages the other person to give you the same kind of information. Or you could show your partner the risk factor list in this book as a way of starting the conversation.

Regardless of how you start the conversation, you will eventually have to get around to discussing each of the risk factors in the chart on page 16. This means asking some pretty personal and rather blunt questions. For many of us, this is the most difficult part of practicing safe sex. But it's also a really important part. Although some people would never tell you about their risk factors if you didn't bring it up, most people won't lie when confronted with a direct question. So, you really do have to ask.

One question that many teen women feel especially embarrassed about asking a male is whether he's ever had any sexual experiences with another male. About 37% of the men in this country have experienced sexual orgasm with another male at some point in their life. Most often this involves some sort of mutual or group masturbation and therefore does not involve any risk for AIDS. However, oral or anal intercourse is not uncommon. So here again, you really do have to ask the question. But don't ask, "Are you bisexual?" People don't think of themselves in terms of these labels. Besides, a male who's had intercourse with another male only once isn't necessarily bisexual, but he could be infected with AIDS. Thus, it is better to ask if he's ever had a sexual experience with another male. You might lead into your question by mentioning the 37% statistic I just quoted, to let him know that you're aware of the fact that this sort of thing is very common.

Both males and females need to ask specifically about past IV drug use. Here again, rather than asking, "Are you an IV drug user?" ask if he or she has ever used needles to take illegal drugs.

What to Do Once You've Found Out

What you do will depend on whether the person has any risk factors, and if so, which ones.

If, to the best of your knowledge, your potential partner doesn't have any risk factors: You can have sex with this person, provided you use a condom and use it properly. However, it's important to remember that people aren't always truthful about these things and they aren't always faithful. So you *must* use a condom!

If your partner refuses to discuss risk factors, will not agree to a monogamous relationship, uses IV drugs, has AIDS, ARC, or positive test results: This person is an unsafe sex partner. It's not safe to have sex with this person, even with a condom. *If the person tries to convince you that it will be safe to have sex as long as you use a condom, don't believe it!*

If a person is, at the present time, an IV drug user, but claims not to be infected because he or she: a) never shares needles with anyone who's infected ("all my buddies are clean!") or b) claims to have had the test, it's still not safe to have sex with that person. Here's why: a) most of the IV drug users currently infected with the AIDS virus have not yet developed symptoms; neither they nor anyone else may have the slightest idea that they're infected; b) a negative

AIDS antibody test is meaningless if a person continues to use IV drugs (see Chapter 4).

If you are deeply in love with a person who uses IV drugs, has AIDS or ARC, or has received a positive antibody test, my heart goes out to you! You need more help than this or any other book can provide. You need face-to-face counseling with a trained AIDS counselor. Call one of the hotline numbers listed on pages 97–100 and ask for a referral to an AIDS counselor in your area.

If the person has used IV drugs in the past, but no longer does so: There's a definite need to be tested before you can consider having sex. But even if the person tests negative, you should be aware of the fact that people who've used drugs in the past often start using again. You will need to discuss this with your partner. You should also consider such things as how long the person has been "clean" (off drugs) and whether he/she regularly attends Narcotics Anonymous or some other support group for former users. If the person hasn't been clean for at least a year and doesn't regularly attend a support group, I personally wouldn't consider this person a safe sex partner, regardless of the test results.

If your partner has had a blood transfusion between 1977 and 1985: As long as your partner did not receive clotting factor concentrates, only had one transfusion, and did not receive more than 3 units of blood, the chances of his or her being infected is very low. Because the risk is low, some experts feel that antibody testing is not necessary in this case. Personally, though, I'd want my potential partner to be tested. After all, why take a chance?

If your partner has had a number of different sex partners or a history of sexually transmitted diseases: Some experts say testing is not necessary unless the person has had *repeated* infections of STDs and/or an *unusually high* number of partners. But, what's an "unusually high" number of partners—4? 8? 28? Does "repeated infections" mean more than 1? 3? 8? You have to use your own judgement here. Of course, to be on the safe side, you can insist on testing.

If the person has any of the other risk factors on the chart: This person is not a safe sex partner until he/she has tested negative for AIDS antibodies on a test taken after 6 months of abstinence from sex and drugs.

If you think that either you or your partner needs AIDS antibody testing, you should consult a trained AIDS counselor beforehand. For more information on AIDS antibody testing and how to obtain proper testing, see pages 100–101.

Safer Sex Guideline #3: Use a Latex Condom Each and Every Time You Have Sex

Condoms (also called "rubbers" or prophylactics) were invented to protect against pregnancy and are placed on the erect penis just before intercourse. A condom fits snugly over the penis in much the same way that a glove fits over a finger and it is held in place by a band of elastic on the lower edge (see Illustration 5). The condom protects the penis from contact with a sex partner's body fluids. And, when the male ejaculates, his semen ("cum") is trapped inside the condom. Thus, condoms help protect both partners against AIDS.

Condoms are made of a thin, elastic material and are available without lubrication or with either a "wet" (jelly) or

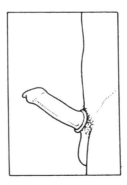

Illustration 5. The Condom Worn Properly Over the Penis

"dry" (silicone powder) lubrication. Some have a plain end; others have a reservoir "tip" (nipple-like tip to collect the semen). There are pink condoms, green condoms, red, white, and blue condoms; ribbed, textured or smooth condoms; straight, contoured or form-fitting condoms; ultra thin and extra-strength, and coming soon—glow-in-the-dark condoms! Try one, try them all—experiment to find the ones you like best.

Use a Condom for All Types of Sex

Any type of intercourse may be capable of spreading the AIDS virus; therefore, you must use a condom for genital and anal sex and also when performing oral sex on a male partner. (For information about oral sex on a female partner, see page 67.)

Use a Latex Condom and Nonoxynol-9

Condoms are made of either latex rubber or natural lambskin. The AIDS virus may be able to pass through the pores in the natural lambskin condom. So, for AIDS prevention, *always use a latex condom.*

When you have anal or genital sex, in addition to using a latex condom, you must also use nonoxynol-9, a spermicidal (sperm-killing) chemical which can kill the AIDS virus. Some brands of wet-lubricated condoms contain nonoxynol-9 and so do most brands of birth control foams, creams, jellies, and sponges. These products, which are also called vaginal contraceptives or vaginal spermicides, are birth control methods which are inserted into the vagina before intercourse to prevent pregnancy (see Illustration 6). For purposes of AIDS prevention, you may use:

- a nonoxynol-9 lubricated latex condom
                      or
- a dry or non-lubricated latex condom *plus* a separate nonoxynol-9 vaginal contraceptive.

There is no scientific evidence to prove that one choice is better than the other. However, the CDC says the condom plus vaginal spermicide combination probably protects you

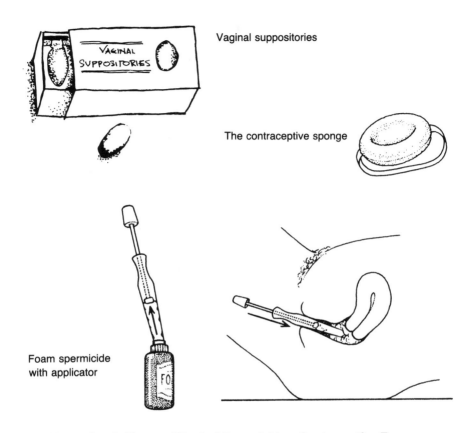

Vaginal suppositories

The contraceptive sponge

Foam spermicide
with applicator

Illustration 6. Types of Vaginal Spermicides: Contraceptive Foams, Creams, Jellies, Gels, and Contraceptive Sponges Foaming tablets (suppositories) are placed in the vagina about 15 minutes before intercourse. They then dissolve, releasing the spermicide.

Contraceptive sponges are shaped like small powder puffs. They are moistened with water to activate the spermicide and then are placed in the top of the vagina.

Special applicators are used to insert the other types of spermicides into the vagina shortly before intercourse. The foams come in aerosol cans, and the applicator is filled by pressing it against the nozzle of the can. The creams, jellies, and gels come in tubes similar to toothpaste tubes; the applicator is attached to the tube and is filled by squeezing on the tube. Once the applicator is filled, the spermicide is inserted by placing the applicator in the vagina and pushing the plunger, releasing the spermicide into the vagina.

better. Studies have shown that contraceptive foam covers the vaginal walls better, and the foaming tablets are especially convenient and easy to use. Many teens prefer the contraceptive sponges because they can be put in place up to 24 hours before intercourse. (The other vaginal spermicides can't be put in more than 30 to 60 minutes ahead of time; consult the instructions that come in the package for exact time.)

How to Use a Condom

Always put the condom on the erect penis *before there's any sexual contact.* The penis must be erect or semi-erect or it will be nearly impossible to put the condom on. Don't "have a little sex first"; the condom absolutely must go on before the penis goes in.

When condoms fail to prevent pregnancy it's usually because the couple *failed to use them at all.* Become a fanatic about using one each and every time you have sex! Condoms are easy to use, but there are all sorts of details to remember. So study the instructions and the following do's and don'ts:

Buy a few and practice before the big moment. Practice makes perfect. In my sex ed classes the boys and the girls practice on bananas—silly, but effective. (Remember, ladies, it's a lot easier to talk to a guy about using condoms if you know what you're talking about!)

Keep a supply handy. Take them along when you go out! (Women, this means you, too!) They can be stored in a wallet or glove compartment for short periods of time, but don't carry condoms loose in a backpack or purse, as this can damage them. Devise a safe container—anything from a funky, tin Band-Aid box to a glamorous antique cigarette case.

Never use petroleum jelly, Vaseline, massage oil, or oil-based lubricants with a condom. These can weaken the latex rubber in a matter of minutes, causing tearing or breaking. Don't use a condom with vaginal medications for yeast infections as they may contain oil.

1. *Open the packet and remove the condom.*

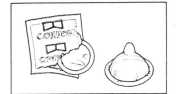

Condoms usually come rolled up in foil or plastic packets. Open the packet and carefully remove the condom. Rough, long, or jagged fingernails or jewelry can damage the condom, so be careful.

2. *Squeeze the air out of the tip and place the condom on the penis.*

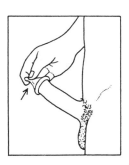

If you are using a brand that doesn't have a built-in reservoir tip (nipple to collect the semen) leave ½″ of space at the top of the condom to allow room for the semen to collect; otherwise, the semen could be forced down the sides of the condom and could leak out at the lower edge.

Holding the tip or the top ½″, place the condom over the end of the erect penis. (If the male is not circumcised, the foreskin should be pulled back first.)

3. *While you're still holding the tip, slowly unroll the condom down the penis.*

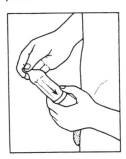

The condom unrolls from the outside and should unroll smoothly. If it doesn't, you've got it inside out, and if you've tugged or pulled on it, throw it out (you may have torn it).

Illustration 7. How to Use a Condom

Illustration 7. How to Use a Condom *(continued)*

4. *Unroll it all the way to the base of the penis and smooth out any wrinkles or air bubbles.*

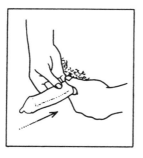

It's important to unroll it all the way; otherwise, sperm may leak out the lower edge. Air bubbles can cause the condom to tear during intercourse, so smooth them out.

5. *Right after ejaculation, hold the condom firmly at the base of the penis and slowly withdraw. Then, discard the condom.*

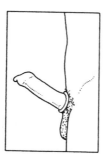

Most men begin to lose their erections soon after ejaculation. As the penis becomes softer and smaller, semen can leak out of the condom or the condom could slip off inside the vagina. So, don't lay there cuddling, withdraw *right* after ejaculation. Condoms aren't family heirlooms and should *never* be reused—throw them out!

Vaginal dryness causes condoms to break or tear; use a water-based lubricant if necessary. Vaginal lubrication is caused by sexual excitement, so don't start intercourse until the vagina is well-lubricated or the condom may tear. If your lovemaking session continues for a long time, dryness may become a problem. If so, use some vaginal spermicide or a water-soluble lubricant (K.Y. Jelly, or better yet, For Play or Pre Pair which contain nonoxynol-9.)

There's a right way and a wrong way to unroll a condom. If you do it the wrong way, the condom won't unroll smoothly for more than perhaps an inch or two. Moreover, the outside of the condom may come into contact with the pre-ejaculatory fluid, which "contaminates" the condom and makes it unusable. So look carefully before you put the condom on.

Don't store condoms in direct sunlight or in places where it gets too hot. Heat and sunlight can deteriorate the rubber.

Don't use a condom that's discolored, brittle, dried-out, if the packet is damaged, torn or already opened, or if the date on the package is more than 2 years ago. Don't open the package until you're ready to use the condom and use a fresh, unopened one each time.

Condoms can be very sexy if you make using them a part of, rather than an interruption to, your love-making. Using condoms *is* a drag if she's lying there, pretending not to notice what's going on, while he politely turns his back and fumbles around under the covers putting the condom on (not to mention the fact that trying to put on a condom when he can't really see what he's doing is awfully awkward for him, and she generally feels pretty stupid just lying there trying to act like nothing's happening).

So, forget all that! Men, put the condom on in front of her—lots of women find this very sexy to watch—and get her involved. You might start by asking her to open the packet. Women, if he turns away, say "Can I help?" or "Show me how to do that." Most men like (love!) to have their partners rub or stroke their penises and most say they're *really* turned on when women put the condom on for them. So, don't hesitate to get it on the act.

If you can get past embarrassment and pretending, using condoms can be a very "sexy" part of your lovemaking. In fact, many couples say that their sex lives actually improved because they started communicating more openly about what they enjoy most during lovemaking.

If condoms (or spermicides) decrease sensitivity for you, try switching brands. Thanks to the new, thinner latex condoms, the old "Using-a-condom-is-like-taking-a-shower-with-your-raincoat-on" saying is not as applicable nowadays. But if this is an issue for you, try a form-fitting condom with a narrow portion that fits closely just behind the head of the penis. Or try placing a dab of water-soluble lubricant in the tip before placing the condom on the penis. (Just a little bit though, or the condom could slip off during intercourse.) Women may prefer a dry lubricated condom or a more concentrated brand of spermicide, with a 5cc instead of a 10cc applicator.

If you find you have questions about using, buying, or storing condoms, you can call 800-4-CONDOM, a toll-free hotline run by the Kimono company (a Japanese condom manufacturer whose high-quality condoms are now available in the United States).

Some Advice for Inexperienced Users

Admitting that it's all new to you can take the pressure off and relax the whole situation. And it's OK to be clumsy or awkward; if you make a mess of the first one, no sweat. Just start again with another one.

For the first few times, many males lose their erection before, during, or after putting a condom on. This is not the end of the world! (Actually, this can happen with or without a condom, and it happens to *all* men now and then.) Getting uptight about this *won't* help. Relax, take a break, hug, cuddle, spend some time learning how to touch each other in ways that feel good. There's always next time, and if you can relax, the penis may become erect again.

Above all, keep your sense of humor. You don't have to be totally solemn or serious about all this. A little humor and laughter can help a lot.

It's Never Too Late to Start Using a Condom

Couples who've been having sex for some time often think there's no point in starting to use condoms because they figure that if one of them is infected, then by now the other one is too. This isn't true. It generally takes many repeated exposures (hundreds, sometimes). However, the longer you continue having sex without condoms, the greater the chances of transmitting any infection. Moreover, if one of you *is* infected, unprotected sex (sex without a condom) may increase chances of developing symptoms and actually coming down with AIDS.

About Oral and Anal Sex

You should not perform oral sex on a male unless he is wearing a condom; the good news is that you needn't use nonoxynol-9. If you want to perform oral sex on a female, you should both have tested negative on a "6-month" AIDS antibody test (see page 54). Or, you can use a rubber dam, a sheet of latex rubber normally used in certain types of dental work, to prevent the exchange of body fluids during oral sex. (However, most people feel the latex is really too thick for this purpose.) If the idea of using rubber dams for oral sex doesn't sound too appealing to you, you're not alone. But what can I tell you? Unprotected oral sex may give you AIDS!

Many experts feel that, even with a condom, anal sex is too risky unless both people have tested negative for AIDS. Other experts feel it's acceptable as long as a heavy-duty condom is used and nonoxynol-9 spermicide or lubricant is first inserted into the rectum.

Using Vaginal Spermicides

These products are easy to use. But mistakes can and do happen, so study the instructions that come in the package carefully, practice first, and keep the following advice in mind:

Don't douche or insert a tampon for at least 8 hours after sex. Douching is not necessary after using any vaginal spermicide. But if you do so, wait at least 8 hours, and don't insert a tampon during that time either. It may absorb the spermicide and leave live sperm in the vagina. (It's OK to use a sanitary napkin, though.)

If more time passes or you have sex a second time, insert a second suppository or applicator or spermicide.

The spermicide gets diluted by vaginal secretions and loses strength over time, so apply a second time if more than 30 minutes have passed since insertion and you are about to have sex again. (This is not necessary with the sponge.)

Always keep a spare package on hand. This is especially important with some brands of foam, as you can't tell ahead of time when the can is almost empty. (If you hear a sputtering sound or the applicator fills more slowly than usual, you need a new can.)

Store spermicides in a cool place. Heat of more than 120 degrees fahrenheit can affect spermicides.

Today's Vaginal Contraceptive Sponges can be put in as much as 24 hours ahead of time. But they often become dislodged, so before you have sex check with your finger to be sure the sponge is still covering the cervix (the firm knob which is the lower portion of the uterus and which protrudes into the top of the vagina). Before you put the sponge in, moisten it with about 2 tablespoons of tap water and squeeze once. Don't use a sponge when you're having your menstrual period. (The blood may cause the sponge to slip out of place.) Leave the sponge in place for at least six hours after intercourse.

Semicid, Encare, and Intercept Contraceptive Tablets or suppositories are convenient, but after inserting the tablet into the vagina, you must wait 10 to 15 minutes before having sex, to give the tablet time to dissolve (see package instructions for exact time).

Buying Condoms and Vaginal Spermicides

You don't need a prescription and anyone, of any age, can buy these products. They're sold in drug stores and in many grocery stores. Planned Parenthood clinics can supply them too and generally have classes to teach teens how to use these products. Condoms are also sold in many convenience stores and vending machines.

There's no need to feel embarrassed buying these products. Sales clerks are used to selling them to people of all ages and both sexes. If you're buying condoms and the salesperson asks you what size you want, he/she means the size of the package (a 3-pack, 6-pack or 12-pack), not the size of the condom. Condoms only come in one size. Some brands tend to run large, though, and some manufacturers make a "snugger fit" that's slightly smaller.

If you have an allergic reaction (skin rash, itch or burning), switch to a different brand.

Make sure that the products you buy contain nonoxynol-9. And always check the manufacturing or expiration date to make sure the products are fresh.

Condoms Alone Are Not Enough Protection

Condoms *definitely* cut down on your chances of getting AIDS, but even with nonoxynol-9 they're not enough protection. Studies of couples using latex condoms to prevent pregnancy have produced failure rates ranging from less than 1% to 22%. Typically, the failure rate is about 10% to 12%. (A failure rate of 10% means that 1 out of 10 women using condoms for one year become pregnant.) There aren't yet any long-term, large-scale studies of how effective condoms are at preventing AIDS. Moreover, the preliminary results of one small study are not encouraging. Eighteen heterosexual couples who continued having sex even after they learned that one of them was infected with AIDS used condoms, in hopes of protecting the uninfected partner. At the end of 18 months, 3 (17%) of the previously uninfected partners had already become infected.

Whatever the effectiveness rate turns out to be, it's clearly not going to be 100%, and it may be a good deal less than that. That's why there are *three* safer sex guidelines, and in addition to using condoms, you must also limit the number of sex partners you have and choose your partners carefully, as discussed earlier.

A Word About Safer Sex, Drugs, and Alcohol

I always say I'm going to be cool, use condoms, not have sex with just anybody, and check a guy out before I jump into bed with him . . . When I get ripped, it all just flies right out the window.

If you're too wasted, you're not going to have sex because you can't get it up. In between sober and totally wasted, that's when it's bad news. You can wind up doing it with someone you hardly know, and you're way past caring if you've got a rubber.

Drugs and alcohol may weaken your immune system making you susceptible to AIDS. And, just about every teen who uses cocaine, Quaaludes, grass, amphetamines, alcohol, or some other drug will tell you that drugs got them into at least one sexual encounter they'd rather just forget about. Chances are they also "forgot" to use a condom, "forgot" about choosing their partners carefully, and "forgot" about limiting the number of partners.

You *don't* want to make decisions about sex when you're drunk or using drugs. Safer sex, drugs and alcohol just don't mix.

As you can no doubt figure out for yourself, one sure-fire way of making sure you don't "forget" about the safer sex guidelines because you're high is to stop getting high altogether. And, if that's what it takes, then that is what you ought to do. After all, this is AIDS we're talking about here, and AIDS kills.

CHAPTER FOUR

Other Types of Transmission and Their Prevention

AIDS CAN ALSO be transmitted by sharing needles used to inject illegal drugs, by infected pregnant women to their babies, and by transfusions of infected blood or blood products. In this chapter, we'll be talking about these types of direct blood-to-blood transmission and also about the prevention of these forms of transmission. Since you've probably heard all sorts of wild rumors about how AIDS is spread, we'll also be talking about mosquitos, toilet seats, and other ways in which AIDS *is not* spread.

Transmission Through Illegal Drug Needles

Sharing needles used to take illegal drugs is the second most common way in which AIDS is spread in this country, and IV drug users are the second largest U.S. group at-risk for AIDS. IV drug use also accounts for a major portion of the AIDS cases in two other risk groups—babies and heterosexual partners:

- 25% of the Americans who've come down with AIDS are IV drug users (of this 25%, 7% are also male homosexuals or bisexuals, while the remainder are male or female heterosexuals)

- 70% of women who've gotten AIDS from a sex partner got it from a male IV drug user
- 70% of the babies born with AIDS have a mother or father—or both—who have used IV drugs

In contrast to the first "wave" of the U.S. epidemic, which primarily struck white, middle-class, gay men, the second wave is hitting poor, minority heterosexuals. Blacks, who account only for 12% of the U.S. population, now account for 26% of the AIDS cases. Hispanics, who make up 6% of the total population, account for 14% of the AIDS cases. This is not to say that whites are unaffected. IV drug use occurs in all races and also at all economic levels.

Just as the "gay" epidemic didn't stay put in New York, San Francisco, etc., this one will travel too. A recent report from Durham, North Carolina, revealed that addicts who tested positive for AIDS antibodies had all shared needles with a "visitor" from New York.

The CDC estimates that there are 1.1 million Americans who currently use IV drugs and that 235,000 of them are already infected. AIDS cases among IV drug users, their sex partners, and their babies will account for an increasing portion of AIDS cases in the coming years. In fact, some experts fear that in the minority communities where poverty, despair, and IV drug use go hand in hand, the epidemic could become nearly as devastating as in Central Africa, where AIDS is expected to wipe out a sizable portion of the population. Indeed, the rate of AIDS infection among pregnant women giving birth in the South Bronx, a borough of New York City, is already within one percentage point of the infection rate among women giving birth in Kinshasa, the capital city of the Central African country of Zaire.

Moreover, IV drug users, many of whom support their drug habits through prostitution, are the pipeline through which the virus may spread into the general heterosexual population. As you know, the experts are arguing about the extent to which the virus will spread among American heterosexuals who don't use drugs and whether there will ever be an epidemic in the general heterosexual population. But it's important to remember that the experts are only arguing about whether we'll be faced with a total catastrophe or "just" a major disaster. In either case, you need to know how to protect yourself personally, and you need to know the facts about what is undoubtedly the major social issue facing our country.

How AIDS Is Spread Through Sharing Drug Needles

It's not the drug itself that causes AIDS. It's sharing the "works" or "rigs"—that is, the needles, syringes, eye droppers, spoons, other containers used to prepare the drug, material used to strain the drug solution, or other equipment used in taking illegal IV drugs. When a person "shoots up" (injects drugs), blood is drawn back up into the needle and syringe. Some of this blood remains on the equipment, and if the person is infected with AIDS, there will be viruses in this blood. Thus, anyone who later uses that equipment can get AIDS. The virus can survive for a short while inside the needle or syringe even if the blood has dried up. So, it's possible to get AIDS from a needle even if quite some time has passed since the infected person used it. Moreover, some of the infected person's blood could remain in the needle or syringe, even if a number of other people had since used it. So, it's not just the person who uses the needle directly after the infected person who can be infected.

Why Addicts Share Dirty Needles

In most states you must have a doctor's prescription to buy needles, and you can be arrested for possession of unprescribed needles. Needles are sometimes sold by drug dealers, but they're expensive and aren't always available. Because it's so difficult to get needles, IV users often share them.

Although you can sterilize needles on your own, it takes time to do so. People who are addicted to IV drugs may start to feel *very, very sick* if they go too long without the drug. By the time they manage to "score" (obtain drugs), they're often too badly in need of a "fix" to take the time to sterilize the needle. Also, using drugs affects your judgment; thus, even if they're not desperately in need of a fix, IV users may

The drugs (heroin, cocaine, "speed," etc.) usually come in powdered or crystal form. They are placed in a "cooker"— a spoon, bottle cap or some other container—and mixed with water. The mixture is then heated to dissolve the drug, and a piece of cotton may be used to strain out any undissolved portion. The solution is then drawn up into a needle and syringe, or eye dropper.

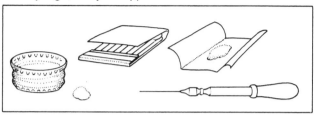

After puncturing the skin, but before injecting the drug, the person draws some blood into the needle and syringe, to make sure that the needle has actually hit a vein. The plunger is then pushed in, injecting the drug into the vein. Often the user will repeat this process to get a better "rush" (high) from the drug. (This also increases the chances of getting or transmitting the AIDS virus.)

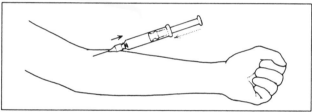

Some of the person's blood *always* remains in the needle and syringe after use. So any AIDS viruses present may be passed on to others who later use the needle or syringe. Flushing the needle out in the cooker can contaminate the cooker with AIDS viruses, as well as the rest of the drug solution and the material used for straining.

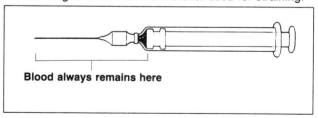

Blood always remains here

Illustration 8. Sharing Equipment Used to Take Illegal Drugs Spreads AIDS

decide not to bother cleaning the needle. Moreover, users often shoot up with "running buddies," friends who score and take drugs together. Cleaning a needle would be considered an insult, as it implies that the buddy isn't "clean" and is infected with the AIDS virus. (It would be kind of like your going to someone's house for dinner and asking him to sterilize the glass and silverware before you ate.) In addition, many IV drug users in New York and other cities in the northeast inject drugs in "shooting galleries," where there generally aren't materials or equipment for sterilizing needles.

Shooting Galleries and the Spread of AIDS

Shooting galleries are usually located in abandoned buildings in the poorer sections of town—in the neighborhoods where drugs are sold on the street. The person who runs the shooting gallery rents out needles and syringes and provides the necessary water and cookers. In some of the larger cities, hundreds of people may be in and out of a shooting gallery in a single day.

It's hard to imagine a better set-up for spreading the AIDS virus to large numbers of people. And not surprisingly, cities with shooting galleries have *very high* rates of AIDS transmission. In New York, for instance, the infection rate among IV drug users is as high as 65% in some areas of the city. On the other hand, in cities such as Los Angeles, where small groups of users meet in residential hotel rooms, homes, or abandoned cars, and the city is too spread out for users to move easily from one gallery to another, the infection rate is more like 5%, though given time, L.A.'s rate will undoubtedly increase.

Prevention Advice for IV Drug Users

To avoid AIDS:

- Stop doing drugs!
- If you can't stop, don't use needles!
- If you must use needles, don't share!
- If you must share needles, clean them first!

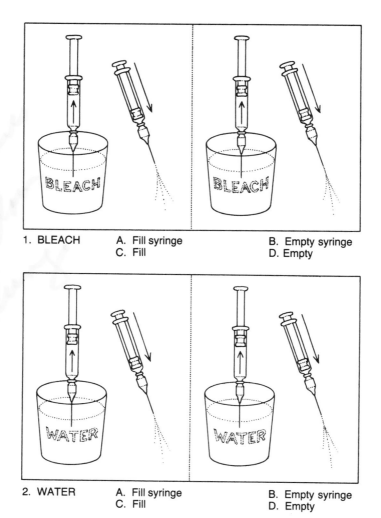

1. BLEACH   A. Fill syringe   B. Empty syringe
                      C. Fill   D. Empty

2. WATER   A. Fill syringe   B. Empty syringe
                      C. Fill   D. Empty

MAKE SURE YOU DON'T SHOOT OR DRINK THE BLEACH!

Illustration 9. How to Clean Needles and Syringes If you use some-body else's "outfit": clean it with bleach, then water. Don't shoot or drink the bleach, though, or you'll get sick! Bleach kills the AIDS virus that gets into used needles. By cleaning them with bleach you will help protect yourself from getting AIDS, and it will not damage the needle.

For information on how to get into a methadone maintenance program or some other program to help you kick your habit, call 1-800-662-4357 (800-662-HELP is a 24-hour, toll-free hotline). These people can also give you information about AIDS antibody testing and about protecting your sex partners from, AIDS. If you have a sex partner who uses IV drugs, see pages 57–58.

Prevention Advice for Non-Users

All IV drug users were once non-users. So, even if you don't use IV drugs, you need to think about drugs and AIDS prevention—to make sure you don't become a needle user. The basic rule is:

> **DON'T USE IV DRUGS,
> NOT EVEN ONCE!**

In fact, it's best to stay away from all illegal drugs and alcohol because they: a) weaken the immune system, making you more susceptible to AIDS; b) have other bad effects on your health—both physical and mental; and c) lead, in some cases, to IV drug addiction. Almost all IV drug users started out on some other drug and "graduated" to using needles. If you are using drugs and need help quitting, call the hotline number listed above.

It's important to know that kids say the main reason they got on drugs in the first place is peer pressure—their friends were doing it. And it was a "friend" who first introduced most IV drug users to needles. In other words, *who* your friends are has a lot to do with whether or not you become a drug user. So check it out.

It's not always easy to resist peer pressure and say "no" to drugs. But if you find yourself in a situation where someone's pressuring you to take drugs, say "no" right away. Be firm, don't apologize, make eye contact, and say the person's name when you refuse. If you look the person right in the eye and use his or her name when you say "no," there's much less chance of the person making fun of you or continuing to pressure you. (Try it, you'll be amazed at how well it works!)

Problems in Preventing Drug-Related AIDS

The above information will help protect you as an individual, but in general, public health officials are not optimistic about the prevention of drug-related AIDS in this society. There are several problems. For one thing, drug use is illegal. This makes it harder for public health officials to reach users with prevention information. Although many of the men in drug abuse treatment programs have demonstrated a willingness to be tested and take steps to avoid infecting others through sex, those who are still using drugs are less likely to identify themselves to authorities by going for AIDS testing.

Female addicts pose a special problem. Most of these women have had very difficult and painful lives. From the time they were just little girls, many were repeatedly beaten and/or raped by their fathers or other family members. Most have never received any help or psychological treatment and, as a result, they tend to think of themselves as worthless human beings and may not care about saving their own lives. Prevention programs designed for these women will need to deal with these issues as well.

Obviously, one way to cut down on drug-related AIDS is to get people off drugs. But treatment is expensive and IV drug users tend to be poor. The waiting list at publicly funded treatment programs is long and a person may have to wait several months or longer. The World Health Organization (WHO) and the President's Commission on AIDS have both recommended that treatment programs be expanded so that any user who wants to quit can receive immediate, free treatment. (This will be less expensive in the long run than the cost of treating AIDS cases among IV users, their babies and their sex partners.) However, the general public is not very sympathetic to, or willing to spend money on, drug users.

Not all addicts will choose to be treated, so the World Health Organization (WHO) has also recommended that governments provide free sterilized needles to stop the spread of AIDS. Many countries have done so, and this has not increased the use of IV drugs in these countries. However, many people in this country fear that passing out needles will encourage more IV drug use. Others object because they feel it would appear that the government is condoning drug use. So far, there are only one or two small, experimental programs in the United States.

Experts are not hopeful of reducing the number of cases in IV drug users any time soon. This also means that the number of babies born with AIDS will continue to increase.

Transmission from Infected Mothers to Their Babies

Among the most tragic manifestations of the HIV[1] epidemic are the infected infants of IV drug abusers. Most of these children die in the first few years of life. Their time on this earth begins with a few months of drug withdrawal in an isolation unit in a hospital and ends after a series of painful illnesses. Few have relatives to visit them while in the hospital. The hardworking nurses, doctors, social workers, and volunteers who staff our acute pediatric care units are father, mother, friend, and teacher to these children.

The President's Commission on AIDS[2]
Interim Report, March 1988

So far, about 700 babies in this country have gotten AIDS from their mothers. Although some of the mothers of these babies got AIDS from blood transfusions or from having sex with a male bisexual, most of these women are IV drug users or the female sex partners of male IV drug users. As the IV drug epidemic grows, so will the number of babies with AIDS.

Babies born to infected mothers develop AIDS symptoms much more quickly than do adults who become infected with the AIDS virus. Though there is one girl who was born to an infected mother and developed AIDS, but remains alive today at the age of nine, the sad fact is that most AIDS babies die or are severely ill by the age of two.

---

[1]HIV stands for human immunodeficiency virus, or the AIDS virus.
[2]The proper name of the commission is actually The Presidential Commission on The Human Immunodeficiency Virus.

Transmission Before, During, and After Birth

Infected women can pass AIDS on to their babies before or during birth because the baby's and the mother's blood are in direct contact during pregnancy and childbirth. There is also one case in which a baby got AIDS from its mother *after* birth. This baby's mother became infected as a result of a blood transfusion she had after her baby was born. Before this woman realized she was infected, she breast-fed her baby and apparently passed the disease on to the child through her breast milk. It is not known exactly how the virus from the mother's breast milk got into the baby's bloodstream. An adult couldn't get AIDS from drinking infected milk. But perhaps a baby's digestive system, which is less developed, can allow this to happen. At any rate, doctors now warn mothers who may be infected with AIDS not to breast-feed their babies.

An infected woman can pass the disease on to her baby, even if she herself doesn't yet have any obvious symptoms of the disease. In fact, in one study, 25% of the women hadn't the faintest idea that they were infected until their babies became sick and it was discovered that their children had AIDS. Even if the mother isn't infected when she first conceives, and only becomes infected after she's already pregnant, her baby could still get AIDS.

The Rate of Transmission

Not all babies born to infected mothers develop AIDS. Experts estimate that anywhere from 30% to 60% of such babies will be born with AIDS. It is not known why some babies born to infected mothers get AIDS while others don't. There have been cases in which a first child was born with AIDS while the second child was not infected, and vice versa. There's even a case in which an infected woman gave birth to twins, and one of the babies was infected, while the other wasn't.

Prevention of Mother-to-Infant Transmission

A couple who is planning to have a baby should be tested for AIDS before she becomes pregnant, unless they are absolutely certain that neither of them could possibly have been exposed to the virus (no transfusion, no drug use, no previous sex partners).

If a woman doesn't find out she has AIDS until after she's already become pregnant, one option is, of course, abortion. However, this is a very personal decision. Some people are absolutely opposed to abortion under any circumstances. But many people feel that abortion is the right choice in this situation. For one thing, if the mother doesn't yet have symptoms, continuing the pregnancy and having the baby may increase her chances of actually coming down with AIDS. Moreover, if the baby does develop AIDS, its short life may be filled with terrible suffering.

Blood and Blood Products

About 3% of the adult and teen AIDS cases in the United States have happened to people who've received transfusions of blood or blood products. This is the one transmission category in which there's some good news to report. Since the spring of 1985, all donated blood in the United States is tested for the AIDS antibody before it's used in transfusions. As a result, the nation's blood supply is much safer, and nowadays there's very little chance of getting AIDS from a transfusion.

Studies have shown that the AIDS virus was not present in the blood supply before 1977, so there's no risk of AIDS from a transfusion given before then. But people who had transfusions between 1977 and March of 1985 may have received contaminated blood. Some of these people have already come down with AIDS and more will do so in the future. However, thanks to AIDS antibody testing, this form of transmission will account for a smaller and smaller portion of U.S. AIDS cases in the future.

The Risk for Hemophiliacs

As I explained in Chapter 1, hemophilia is a clotting disorder. For people with hemophilia, even a slight bump or bruise can cause uncontrollable internal bleeding. The disease is inherited (passed on in families, from one generation to the next) and is almost always passed on to male children, though there are some female hemophiliacs. There are also other less common clotting disorders, e.g., von Willebrand's disease. Like hemophilia, these other disorders are treated with a blood product called clotting factor concentrate, which is made by taking a small amount of clotting factor from the blood of many, many different donors. A person with a clotting disorder may require a number of transfusions each year; thus, people with clotting disorders may be exposed to the blood of thousands of different donors. It's not surprising, then, that about 70% of the Americans with severe hemophilia and 35% of those with the milder form of the disease have already been infected. Fortunately, hemophilia is a rare disease, so altogether there are only about 10,000 infected hemophiliacs in the United States. Since all donated blood is now tested for AIDS and clotting factor concentrate is treated by heat, the risk to hemophiliacs has also been practically eliminated.

Risk for Others Who Received Transfusions in the Past

Among other Americans who received transfusions between 1977 and 1985, the chances of having received infected blood are greater for those in cities such as New York, San Francisco, Los Angeles, and Washington, D.C., where AIDS is the most widespread. The risk is also greater for people who received multiple transfusions or several units of blood during a single transfusion.

However, if you received a transfusion during those years, you should know that as long as you didn't receive clotting factors, the chances that you received infected blood are very small. Between 1977 and 1985, 20–35 million Americans received transfusions, but experts estimate that only about 24,000 to 45,000 of these people received infected blood. About 60% of them have already died, either from the operation that caused them to need the transfusion or from other causes not related to AIDS. That leaves roughly 10,000–20,000 people still alive who were infected from transfusions. So, even if you did receive a transfusion between 1977 and 1985, the odds are in your favor.

Some hospitals are participating in "look back" programs to trace and test people who may have received infected transfusions. However, many hospitals have chosen not to participate in these programs. Although the odds of being infected are small, the CDC recommends that all people who received transfusions between 1977 and 1985 have an AIDS antibody test.

The Present Risk

Although the risk of getting AIDS from a transfusion has been greatly reduced, it has not been completely eliminated. One recent study indicated that as many as 460 people per year were still becoming infected through transfusions. The problem is that AIDS antibody tests can't always spot infected blood, usually because the donor has become infected only recently and hasn't yet developed enough antibodies to show up on the test. (Remember, it can take up to six months to develop enough antibodies to show up on the test.)

However, in addition to testing the blood, other steps are now being taken to cut down on the chances of an infected person donating blood:

- Before people give blood, they must read a pamphlet that describes AIDS, lists the symptoms, and explains that certain people—for example, those who've used IV needles to take illegal drugs, and males who've had sex with other males—may be infected and should not donate blood.
- Then, donors are asked, both out loud and in writing, a series of questions to see if they might be infected. If so, they aren't allowed to give blood.
- Since some donors might be too embarrassed to give honest answers, there is a box on the form that people can check to indicate that their blood should be used "for research purposes only, not for transfusions."
- Since some people might be worried about others seeing that they've checked the box, donors are also given a phone number they can call later to indicate that their blood should not be used. They don't even have to give their name, just the identification number on their blood donor card.

Between these steps and the AIDS antibody testing, the Public Health Service's best estimate is that, nowadays, a person who receives an "average transfusion" (about three units of blood) probably has only about a 1-in-34,000 chance of getting infected blood.

A Note About Blood Donation

Disposable equipment is used for collecting blood, so there's never been any risk of getting AIDS from *donating* blood. If a donor's blood does test positive for AIDS antibodies, the donor is notified and given personal counseling. However, if you have any reason at all to think you may have been infected and you want antibody testing, DO NOT DONATE BLOOD as a way of getting free testing! This endangers other people's lives. A single unit donated by an infected adult can, theoretically, infect 16 babies (because a baby needing a blood transfusion usually requires only $\frac{1}{16}$ of a unit)! If you want free testing, go to an alternate testing site (see page 100).

Other Types of Transmission: Rumors, Fears, and Facts

In Chapter 1, I explained that the rumors about AIDS being transmitted through casual contact just aren't true, and I told you why scientists are sure that AIDS can't be spread through casual contact. In this section, we'll be discussing still more rumors and also the real facts about the proven forms of transmission.

As of June 1988, the only proven cases of AIDS infection that have not been attributed to sexual intercourse, IV drug needles, transfusions, or being born to an infected mother are:

- A few people who became infected after organ transplant operations. Nowadays, donated organs are first tested for antibodies, so the chances of this happening are now greatly reduced.
- A small number of women who received infected semen during artificial insemination, a procedure often used to help the wives of infertile men become preg-

nant. Here again, donated semen is now tested for AIDS antibodies, so there is little chance of this happening anymore.

- A small number of healthcare workers who had needle-stick accidents or contact between "wet" skin and infected body fluids through work-related accidents. Most of them worked with AIDS patients or in a job that involved taking or handling large amounts of blood and, on one or more occasions, had accidentally stuck themselves with a needle in the course of their work. For example, one was a nurse who had stuck herself at least twice while drawing blood from an AIDS patient.

- A few healthcare workers who had some sort of skin infection or a break in their skin and became infected with the AIDS virus after being exposed to large amounts of infected blood.

- 2 healthcare providers who had taken care of AIDS patients over a *long* period of time and *often* had close contact with infected blood, feces, and/or urine. Though neither specifically recalled having infections, open sores, or cuts on their skin, they had not worn gloves when handling these body fluids, and they didn't always wash their hands afterward.

- 2 research lab workers whose jobs included handling AIDS viruses concentrated to more than a 1000 times the normal strength. Though one worker doesn't remember any cuts, here again, proper safety precautions weren't followed.

- 1 healthcare worker who tested positive for AIDS antibodies, and whose written form indicated he had no risk factors, but who could not be located for questioning.

AIDS in Healthcare Workers

It's important to understand the real facts about the healthcare worker cases mentioned above, for these cases have given many people mistaken ideas about AIDS transmission and have started many false rumors. Moreover, if you understand these cases, you'll also understand the basic principles of AIDS transmission. So, lets take a closer look at some of these cases.

Needle-stick cases. There are many thousands of doctors, nurses, lab technicians, and other healthcare workers in this country, and there are tens of thousands of needle-stick accidents each year. Yet, only a dozen or so health workers, reportedly, have gotten AIDS in this way.

Normally, it takes being exposed to large amounts of virus directly into the bloodstream (as in transfusions) or repeated exposures of small amounts of virus (as in IV drug users) to cause infection. But we do know that a few people have become infected after only one time of having sex with an infected person, and these needlestick accidents seem to confirm that *some people are especially susceptible to AIDS*.

Cases in which workers were exposed to blood. Hearing about these cases has given many people the mistaken idea that anyone who has a cut or break in the skin and is exposed to infected body fluids is likely to get AIDS. But there are two things you have to know about these cases. First of all, these workers were exposed to *large* amounts of blood. In one case, for example, malfunctioning equipment caused infected blood to spray all over the room and all over the healthcare worker operating the equipment.

Unless the blood is injected directly into the bloodstream, it's unlikely that exposure to small amounts of blood (or any other infected body fluid) could cause infection because *the number of AIDS viruses per drop of blood is very low*. There are only one to one hundred AIDS viruses per milliliter (about 5 drops) of blood. In comparison, a milliliter of blood from the body of a person who has hepatitis B (a disease which is also caused by a virus that lives in human body fluids) contains 100 million to 1 billion hepatitis viruses.

The second thing you should know is that many of these workers had skin breaks because they had skin *infections or diseases*. In fact, they had chronic (long-time) skin problems. For example, one was a nurse with a skin condition known as eczema that caused her hands to be red, raw, and chapped.

When a person has such a condition, large numbers of infection-fighting white blood cells of the immune system called lymphocytes rush to the scene of the infection. As long as the condition persists, there will be large numbers of lymphocytes in the area. As it so happens, these are the very cells that the AIDS virus especially likes to infect. Because this nurse and these other healthcare workers had chronic skin infections, they not only had skin breaks, but also lots of lymphocytes, in the area of the break—a perfect set-up for the AIDS virus!

The two cases in which healthcare providers became infected. Remember, both these people had regular close contact with infected blood, feces, and/or urine. Neither of these people remembers having a skin infection, a cut, or any other skin break. But they had not worn gloves when handling these body fluids, and they didn't necessarily wash their hands afterward. Moreover, these people cared for AIDS patients over *long* periods of time. For instance, one was a nurse who cared for her own baby after he developed AIDS from having a blood transfusion. Without the protection of gloves, she drew blood from the infant, inserted various feeding tubes into the child's body, changed his diapers during his many bouts of diarrhea. If this nurse had only been exposed to the virus once or twice, then a simple, uninfected skin break probably wouldn't have led to AIDS.

Exposure Through Skin Breaks: Blood Brothers, Razors, Toothbrushes, Pierced Ears, and Acupuncture and Tattoo Needles

What if two guys were punching each other out and had bruises and cuts and their bleeding cuts get pressed against each other? What if you cut your finger and then you were at the scene of a car accident and got someone's blood on your cut finger?

The kids in my class ask these sorts of questions all the time. I explain that it would be highly unlikely for a person to get AIDS in such situations. Still, a good general rule to follow is: Avoid doing *anything* that would put an open sore, cut, rash, or any break in your skin in contact with another person's body fluids. Students often ask about the following sorts of situations:

Blood brothers. Sometimes kids will prick their fingers to make a drop of blood and then press their fingers together as a pledge of friendship, and there've been some rumors about AIDS being passed on in this way. The fact is that no one has ever gotten AIDS in this way, and it's not very likely that anyone will. For one thing, there are really very few kids in this country who are infected with AIDS; it's mostly older people who are infected. So, even if you did do this, it's unlikely that the kid you did it with would be infected. Still, to be on the safe side, you shouldn't do this sort of thing.

Razors and toothbrushes. There are no known cases of AIDS passed on in this way, and it has been studied in the households of AIDS patients. But people do bleed while brushing and they do cut themselves while shaving. So, though these aren't very likely ways of getting AIDS, you should not use another person's razor or toothbrush.

Pierced ears. Pierced earlobes sometimes bleed a bit. Moreover, there's frequently a low-grade infection of some type present, so there's all those white blood cells available for the AIDS virus to infect. If you've shared earrings in the past, I wouldn't stay up nights worrying about it, but I wouldn't borrow or lend them in the future.

Acupuncture and tattoo needles. There are no proven cases of persons being infected with AIDS in these ways. However, I would want to make *very* sure that tattoo needles were sterilized and that disposable acupuncture needles were used if I were having either of these procedures done.

Human Bites and Tears

Since the AIDS virus can live in saliva, no one can say that it is absolutely impossible to get AIDS from a human bite. However, a number of doctors, nurses, and other people have been bitten by AIDS patients, and *none* of these people has actually become infected. The reason they didn't become infected probably has to do with the fact that so few viruses are found in saliva, too few to cause an infection. Also, recent research indicates that a chemical found in saliva may inactivate the AIDS virus. Besides, only some infected people have viruses in their saliva and, even when they do, the number of viruses is very small. So bites are just not a very likely means of transmission.

You'd be even less likely to get AIDS from someone spitting on your scratched knee or from putting your cut finger in someone's mouth. (Obviously, though, it's not a good idea to put your fingers in someone else's mouth or to let someone lick your cuts, though really, this is more because of the danger of other infections than because of AIDS.)

The virus is also found in tears, but only in very small numbers. So, you needn't worry about getting AIDS from someone's tears.

Mosquitos and Other Insects

The rumor that mosquitos could pass on AIDS began some years back when an unusually high number of cases were found in a town in Florida where mosquitos are common. But it turned out that these cases were caused by people sharing IV drug needles or having sex with an infected person, not by mosquitos.

Although it's true that malaria is spread by mosquitos, the malaria germ actually becomes part of the mosquito's life cycle. The AIDS virus does not, and experts feel very sure that mosquitos do not spread AIDS. For one thing, even if an insect bit you immediately after biting an infected person, it's unlikely that the tiny amount of blood that might be left on the stinger would have enough viruses in it to actually cause infection. Besides, if insects like mosquitos could transmit the disease, there'd be lots of cases of AIDS in areas of the country that have lots of mosquitos; however, this isn't the case.

Cats and Other Animals

You may have heard that cats can carry the AIDS virus. Although there is a virus that can affects cats and that comes from the same general family of viruses as the AIDS virus, cats definitely don't carry the AIDS virus. You can't get AIDS from a cat or any other animal.

Food

When I tell the kids in my class that you can't get AIDS from eating food prepared by someone with AIDS, they want to know, "What if the infected person spit in your food or accidentally got cut and bled into your food?" You'd still be safe. The AIDS virus doesn't live in or on food. Moreover, the virus doesn't enter your bloodstream through the digestive tract. So, even in the unlikely event of someone spitting or bleeding into your food, you wouldn't get AIDS.

Toilet Seats

You really needn't worry about toilet seats. One of the kids in my class wanted to know whether you could get AIDS if you had a flea bite on your rear end and sat on a toilet seat that had a few drops of urine splashed on it. I explained that it's true that urine may occasionally contain small amounts of the virus. But, even if there were a flea bite or some other break in the skin, it's unlikely that this sort of contact with infected urine would transmit AIDS. However, no one can say that it would be absolutely impossible to get AIDS in this way, and, of course, you should always wipe off a toilet seat that seems dirty. But, on the whole, I'd say you should spend about as much time worrying about getting AIDS from a toilet seat as you do worrying about being flattened by a herd of stampeding elephants.

CHAPTER FIVE

Joining the Fight Against AIDS

IN THIS BOOK we've talked about what you can do to protect yourself against AIDS and help stop the spread of this disease. Here, in these closing pages, I'd like to talk about some of the other ways in which you can help in the fight against AIDS.

Educate your friends and classmate about AIDS. You can do this on a personal level by talking to your friends about this disease, telling them what you've learned about AIDS prevention, and lending them this book.

You can educate your classmates by bringing the topic of AIDS up in classroom "current events" discussions. You could also arrange with your teacher to show an AIDS film or video (see pages 95–86) or to invite guest speakers to discuss AIDS from a medical, social or political point of view (for example, a knowledgeable doctor, a local public health official, a representative from a gay community organization, a person with AIDS, a local U.S. congressman, or a state government official).

Co-ordinate an AIDS Awareness Week at your school or college. Begin by getting support from the administration, i.e., your school principal or college president. Approach other school or campus groups about co-sponsoring the event. Ask the drama class or theatre department to stage a play or skit about AIDS. Arrange for the school library or campus book store to feature AIDS books and journals. Provide the student newspaper with material for a series of articles on AIDS. Order free pamphlets from your state health department. Events during the week might include showing AIDS films and videos, guests lecturers, question and answer sessions, group discussions, and public debates. The section that follows, "For Further Information," lists pamphlets, films, videos and useful groups to contact if you decide to organize an AIDS Awareness Week.

Volunteer your time. There are more than 400 community-based organizations that provide AIDS-related services —raising funds for AIDS research; shopping, cooking, or doing household chores for people with AIDS; running AIDS information hotlines; operating AIDS testing, counseling, and medical care clinics; hugging and cuddling babies on AIDS hospital wards; educating the public about the epidemic; delivering meals-on-wheels; and lobbying for AIDS legislation (to mention just a few of the valuable services these groups provide). You can help in lots of ways, even if it's just by stuffing envelopes and licking stamps. So get in touch with an AIDS organization in your area and find out how you can help (see pages 97–100). You can also contact the National AIDS Network, 1012 Fourteenth Street, N.W., Suite 601, Washington, D.C. 20005, (202) 347-0390 for information on programs in your community.

The PWA Memorial Bracelet Program. Sponsored by Mothers of AIDS Patients (MAP) and the Public War on AIDS Endowment Fund, the PWA Bracelet Program was created to establish a national symbol of unity in the war against AIDS, and to honor the thousands of men, women and children who have fallen to this disease. The metal bracelets are designed for both men and women and come in gold or silver color. Each memorial bracelet bears the name, age, and date of death of someone who has died of AIDS. The bracelets are available for a donation of $10 or more; the proceeds help provide funding for MAP, the PWA Endowment Fund, and other organizations that assist and support people with AIDS and their families. For more information, or to order a bracelet, call 800-248-0465 (toll free); or, if you live in California, call 213-933-0093.

FOR FURTHER
INFORMATION

THE INFORMATION IN this book is based on the most current research available at the time it was written; however, scientists are making new discoveries all the time. If you're concerned that something in this book isn't completely up-to-date or you have questions that aren't answered here, you can call the 24-hour National AIDS Hotline, toll-free. For a three-minute recorded tape about AIDS in English or Spanish, call (800) 342-AIDS (that's 800-342-2437). If you wish to speak to an AIDS counselor directly, the 24-hour, toll-free hotline number to call is (800) 342-7514.

General Information About AIDS

In addition to the AIDS hotlines, there are a number of organizations that provide printed or audiovisual materials about AIDS, including:

The U.S. Public Health Service provides a number of AIDS information services and materials, including free copies of the *Surgeon General's Report On Acquired Immune Deficiency Syndrome*. This pamphlet is available in English or Spanish and may be obtained by calling, toll-free, 800-342-7514.

ETR Associates, Network Publications, P.O. Box 1830, Santa Cruz, California, 95061-1830 is an excellent source of educational materials for parents, teachers, and teens on AIDS, sexuality, and drug abuse. Write for a free copy of their general catalog and their special AIDS catalog. The pamphlets listed on pages 95–96 and 101 that are marked with an asterisk * are available from Network Publications. Multiple copies are available at low cost and single copies are available free of charge. Up to 20 different pamphlets may be requested. For every set of 6 (or fewer) different pamphlets requested, send a pre-stamped ($.65), pre-addressed, business-size (4" × 9½") envelope. On the back of the envelope write both the names and the title numbers of the free pamphlets you are requesting.

The Red Cross publishes the "Latest Facts About AIDS" pamphlets. Titles in this series include: *AIDS, Sex and You: Facts About AIDS and Drug Abuse;* and *Gay and Bisexual Men and AIDS.* These are free, except for postage if you order a large quantity. Call your local Red Cross for information on obtaining these materials or contact the American Red Cross AIDS Education Office, 1730 D Street, N.W., Washington, D.C. 20006, 202-737-8300. The Red Cross also has a number of AIDS films and videos which can be borrowed free of charge by contacting Modern Talking Picture Service, 5000 Park Street North, St. Petersburg, Florida 33709, 813-541-5763.

The San Francisco AIDS Foundation Materials Distribution Dept., 333 Valencia Street, 4th Floor, San Francisco, California 94103, publishes very explicit prevention materials for gays and drug users, materials specially designed for women and minority groups, as well as excellent books and pamphlets for people with AIDS, ARC, or positive antibody tests. Many of their materials are available in Spanish. Write for their free catalog.

Gay Men's Health Crisis Box 274, 132 West 24th Street, New York, New York 10011, also publishes very frank pamphlets on prevention for gays and drug users, as well as excellent, low-cost pamphlets on all aspects of AIDS for gays, minorities, and women. Many of its publications are available in Spanish and some are available in Mandarin Chinese. Their *INFO PACK* contains several pamphlets and is free, as is their *GAY INFO PACK* (includes all the pamphlets in the *INFO PACK*, plus some even franker pamphlets written for gay men, using "street language"). Send a self-addressed, stamped envelope (and it never hurts to send at least a dollar or two to cover printing costs).

AIDS Pamphlets, Films, and Videos for Teens

There are a number of AIDS pamphlets and audiovisual materials aimed at teens, many of which are available for free or at low cost.

Some of these are listed below. Unfortunately, most AIDS prevention materials discuss only abstinence and condoms. They often fail to mention nonoxynol-9 or the fact that condoms are not 100% effective, and they frequently don't discuss the other two safer sex guidelines at all. So, if you use these materials, be sure to stress these points.

Pamphlets

AIDS: Am I At Risk?—A Checklist for Modern Lovers, from ETR Associates, title #171.*

AIDS—Think About It, from ETR Associates, title #162 (available in Spanish).*

Can We Talk?, for sexually active male teens, available from the S.F. AIDS Foundation, cost $.30. Also ask for the latest issue of their condom newsletter, cost $2.00.

Condoms and STD, from ETR Associates, title #173.*

Deciding About Sex: The Choice to Abstain, from ETR Associates, title #138.*

Talking With Your Partner About Safer Sex, from ETR Associates, title #159.*

Teens & AIDS: Why Risk It?, from ETR Associates, title #161.*

What Do We Know About AIDS?, from ETR Associates, title #111.*

What Is Safer Sex?, from ETR Associates, title #160.*

What Women Should Know About AIDS, from ETR Associates, title #136.*

What You Should Know About The AIDS Antibody Test, from ETR Associates, title #172.

Films and Videos

AIDS, 18 minutes, available in film or videotape format. Hosted by Ally Sheedy, this film is aimed at junior and senior high school students. For information on purchase or rental, call or write Walt Disney Educational Media Co., Consumer Service Division, 10316 N.W. Prairie View Road, Kansas City, MO, 64153-9990 or call (800) 423-2555.

Answers About AIDS, 16 minutes, available only in video format. I have only seen the Red Cross film for adults, *AIDS: Beyond*

Fear; however, it's good, as are all the Red Cross materials. So, presumably, this film, which is aimed at teenagers, is too. And it has the great advantage of being free. Contact Modern Talking Picture Service (address on page 94) for information about borrowing the film.

Sex, Drugs, & AIDS, 18 minutes, available in film or video format. Hosted by Rae Dawn Chong, this is an excellent film for a teenage audience. Since the film only shows girls discussing condom use, it's important to emphasize that AIDS prevention is the male's, as well as the female's, responsibility. Another version of this film, entitled *The Subject Is AIDS*, emphasizes abstinence and also incorporates other changes that make it suitable for a junior high school audience. For information regarding purchase or rental of either film, write to O.D.N. Productions, 74 Varick Street, Suite 304, New York, New York 10013 or call (212) 431-1604. There's also a book that contains stills and captions from the first film (*Sex, Drugs & AIDS*, by Oralee Wachter, New York: Bantam Books, 1987).

AIDS Pamphlets for Parents and Educators

These pamphlets are designed to help parents and teachers deal with this difficult topic.

AIDS and Children: Information for Parents of School-Age Children, available for free from the Red Cross.

AIDS and Children: Information for Teachers and School Officials, available for free from the Red Cross.

How to Talk to Your Teens and Children About AIDS, produced by the National PTA. Single copy $.20; $15.00 for 100 copies. To order, write to AIDS Brochure, 700 N. Rush Street, Chicago, Illinois 60611 or call (312) 787-0977.

How to Talk to Your Children About AIDS, produced by the Sex Information and Education Council of the United States. The first 2 copies are free; up to 50 copies are $.60 each. To order, write to New York University, SIECUS Library, 5th Floor, 32 Washington Place, New York, NY 10003.

Talking With Your Child About AIDS, from ETR Associates, title #169.*

Talking With Your Teenager About AIDS, from ETR Associates, title #170.*

Your Child and AIDS, $.90 from S.F. AIDS Foundation, address given on page 94.

AIDS Hotlines

In addition to the National AIDS hotline numbers given above, a number of cities and some states also operate hotlines. These numbers are listed below (*800* numbers are toll-free).

Alabama
Birmingham — 800-445-3741

Alaska
Entire State — 800-478-AIDS

Arizona
Tucson — 602-326-AIDS

Arkansas
Little Rock — 501-374-5503

California
Costa Mesa — 714-534-0862
Fresno — 209-264-2437
Los Angeles — 213-876-AIDS
San Diego — 619-543-0300
San Francisco — 800-FOR-AIDS
San Rafael — 415-457-2437
Elsewhere in California — 800-922-2437

Colorado
Denver — 303-837-0166

Connecticut
Hartford — 203-236-4431
New Haven — 203-624-2437

Delaware
Entire state — 302-652-6776

District of Columbia
Washington — 202-332-5295

Florida
Miami — 305-634-4636
West Palm Beach — 305-582-4357
Elsewhere in Florida — 800-325-5371

Georgia
Atlanta — 800-551-2728

Idaho
Boise — 208-345-2277

Illinois

Chicago	312-908-9191
Elsewhere in Illinois	800-AID-AIDS

Indiana

Indianapolis	317-257-HOPE

Iowa

Entire state	800-445-AIDS

Kansas

Topeka	800-247-7499

Kentucky

Louisville	502-637-4342

Louisiana

New Orleans	800-992-4379

Maine

Portland	800-851-AIDS

Maryland

Baltimore	800-638-6252

Massachusetts

Entire state	800-235-2331

Michigan

Detroit	313-567-1640
Grand Rapids	616-956-9009

Minnesota

Minneapolis	800-248-AIDS

Mississippi

Jackson	601-353-7611

Missouri

Kansas City	816-561-8784
St. Louis	314-531-7400

Montana

Billings	406-252-1212

Nebraska

Omaha	402-342-4233

Nevada

Las Vegas	702-369-6162

New Hampshire
Concord, Manchester   603-880-6560

New Jersey
New Brunswick   201-596-0767

New Mexico
Entire state   800-858-2437

New York
Albany   518-445-AIDS
Bridgehampton   516-385-AIDS
Buffalo   716-847-AIDS
New York   718-596-4781
                                   212-807-6655
Rochester   716-232-4430
Syracuse   315-875-AIDS

North Carolina
Asheville   704-252-7489
Charlotte   704-333-2437
Greensboro   919-275-1654
Raleigh   919-733-7301
Wilmington   919-675-9222

Ohio
Cincinnati   513-352-3139
Cleveland   216-621-0766
Columbus   614-224-0411
Toledo   419-243-9351

Oklahoma
Oklahoma City   405-525-AIDS

Oregon
Portland   800-777-AIDS

Pennsylvania
Philadelphia   215-732-AIDS
Pittsburgh   412-363-2437

Rhode Island
Providence   401-277-6502

South Carolina
Columbia   803-777-2273

South Dakota
Sioux Falls   605-332-4599

Tennessee
Knoxville	615-523-AIDS
Nashville	615-385-AIDS

Texas
Austin	512-458-AIDS
Dallas	214-559-AIDS
Houston	713-524-2437

Utah
Salt Lake City	801-486-2437

Vermont
Burlington	802-863-2437

Virginia
Richmond	804-358-6343

Washington
Seattle	206-323-1229

Wisconsin
Milwaukee	800-334-2437

Information About AIDS Antibody Testing

AIDS antibody testing is available at public health clinics, hospitals, doctors' offices, and other locations. Testing is usually free at public health clinics; elsewhere fees range from $20 to $150. Before testing, you should receive counseling about the many legal, social, and emotional issues involved in AIDS antibody testing. Although medical information is usually confidential, some states have laws which require that the names of people who test positive be reported to public health departments. The courts can also require doctors and hospitals to release medical information.

Anonymous testing is available in many places. (You don't give your name and are assigned a code number known only to you. Test results are posted by code number.) Anonymous testing is available for free at "alternative testing sites," and some local public health departments and private clinics also offer anonymous testing. Call your local health department, community AIDS hotline, or the national AIDS hotline for the location of the nearest alternative testing site or anonymous testing center that offers counseling as well as the testing itself.

The following pamphlets will help you to understand the pros and cons of testing:

AIDS Antibody Testing at Alternative Test Sites, available from the San Francisco AIDS Foundation at the address on page 94.

If Your Test for Antibody to the AIDS Virus Is Positive . . ., available free from the Red Cross. Call your local chapter or write to national headquarters at the address on page 94.

What You Should Know about the AIDS Antibody Test, available from ETR Associates, Network Publications, title #172.*

INDEX

LYNDA MADARAS BOOKS FOR PRE-TEENS AND TEENS (AND THEIR FAMILIES)
Available in both gift hardcover and trade paperback

Lynda Madaras' four growing-up books are highly recommended by reviewers, doctors, educators, librarians, and readers for their tone ("Conversational, matter-of-fact, honest" — *Washington Post*) and coverage ("Madaras tackles some of the hardest subjects with the aim of provoking discussion rather than conveying her own point of view" — *Kirkus Reviews*).

See next page for information about these books and how to obtain them.

THE WHAT'S HAPPENING TO MY BODY? BOOK FOR GIRLS,
New Edition
A Growing-Up Guide for Parents and Daughters
Lynda Madaras with Area Madaras
Foreword by Cynthia Cooke, M.D.
288 pages; 44 drawings; bibliography; index.

THE WHAT'S HAPPENING TO MY BODY? BOOK FOR BOYS,
New Edition
A Growing-Up Guide for Parents and Sons
Lynda Madaras with Dane Saavedra
Foreword by Ralph I. Lopez, M.D.
272 pages; 34 drawings; bibliography; index.

Newly revised and updated, these two bestselling puberty education
books for 8- to 15-year-olds, their parents, and other concerned adults
now include information appropriate for this age level about AIDS,
other sexually transmitted diseases (STDs), and birth control.

THE WHAT'S HAPPENING? WORKBOOK FOR GIRLS
Lynda Madaras and Area Madaras
128 pages

The latest edition to Newmarket's parenting/teen-care library.
Quizzes, checklists, and innovative exercises encourage expression
of feelings about a young girl's changing body.

LYNDA MADARAS' GROWING-UP GUIDE FOR GIRLS
Lynda Madaras with Area Madaras
224 pages; 30 drawings; bibliography.

The companion workbook/journal to *The What's Happening to My
Body? Book for Girls* will help pre-teens and teens further explore
their changing bodies and their relationships with parents, teachers,
and friends; complete with space to record personal experiences.

LYNDA MADARAS TALKS TO TEENS ABOUT AIDS
An Essential Guide for Parents, Teachers, and Young People
Lynda Madaras
Foreword by Constance Wofsy, M.D.
128 pages; 9 drawings; resource guide; index.

Everything teens need to know to protect themselves against AIDS.
Written especially for 14- to 19-year olds (whether sexually active or
not), this book separates the facts from the rumors, explains the sexual
transmission of AIDS and its prevention (including comprehensive
information on abstinence and safe sex), and more.

LYNDA MADARAS BOOKS FOR PRE-TEENS AND TEENS (AND THEIR FAMILIES)

Order from your local bookstore or write to:

Newmarket Press, 18 East 48th Street, New York, N.Y. 10017 (212) 832-3575.

Please send me the following books by Lynda Madaras:

THE WHAT'S HAPPENING TO MY BODY? BOOK FOR GIRLS

_____ copies at $16.95 each (gift hardcover)

_____ copies at $9.95 each (trade paperback)

THE WHAT'S HAPPENING TO MY BODY? BOOK FOR BOYS

_____ copies at $16.95 each (gift hardcover)

_____ copies at $9.95 each (trade paperback)

THE WHAT'S HAPPENING? WORKBOOK FOR GIRLS

_____ copies at $9.95 each (trade paperback)

LYNDA MADARAS' GROWING-UP GUIDE FOR GIRLS

_____ copies at $16.95 each (gift hardcover)

_____ copies at $9.95 each (trade paperback)

LYNDA MADARAS TALKS TO TEENS ABOUT AIDS

_____ copies at $14.95 each (gift hardcover)

_____ copies at $6.95 each (trade paperback)

For postage and handling, add $2.00 for the first book, plus $1.00 for each additional book. Please allow 4-6 weeks for delivery. Prices and availability subject to change.

I enclose a check or money order, payable to Newmarket Press, in the amounts of $ _____ .

(NYS residents please add sales tax.)

Name _____

Address _____

City/State/Zip _____

Organizations, clubs, firms, and other groups may qualify for special discounts on quantity purchases of these titles. For further information, or for a copy of our catalog, please write or phone Newmarket Press at the address given above.   BOB 078801